Congenital Heart Disease

Lisa Bergersen · Susan Foerster · Audrey C.
Marshall · Jeffery Meadows
Editors

Congenital Heart Disease

The Catheterization Manual

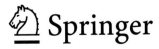 Springer

Editors

Lisa Bergersen
Department of Cardiology
Children's Hospital Boston
Boston, MA 02115

Susan Foerster
Washington University in St. Louis
St. Louis, MO 63110

Audrey C. Marshall
Department of Cardiology
Children's Hospital, Boston
Boston, MA 02115

Jeffery Meadows
Division of Pediatric Cardiology
University of California at San Francisco
San Francisco, CA 94143

ISBN: 978-0-387-77291-2   e-ISBN: 978-0-387-77292-9
DOI 10.1007/978-0-387-77292-9

Library of Congress Control Number: 2007940923

springer.com

Contents

A brief history of the Fellows' Manual
The Fellows' Manual originated many years ago as an introductory collection of advice and papers compiled by senior pediatric cardiology fellows at Children's Hospital Boston. The original "editions" were quite informal, consisting of loosely organized, hand-typed case examples and copied articles, which were passed down year after year from senior cardiology fellows to new first-year fellows as they entered the "cath lab" for the first time. The spirit of the manual remains the same. As written in the manual's 1999 in-house "edition":

> *...These essays are intended to complement the existing didactic programs and structure of the catheterization lab, not to replace them. Although often very detailed, the essays obviously are neither exhaustive nor authoritative, and should be viewed as your personal "lecture notes," to be updated and amended by you on an ongoing basis based upon your experience and study. In other words, the essays per se do not constitute quotable literature. For this reason, select articles ... have been included at the end of the manual....*

Layout
For simplicity, this manual is broken up into two sections. The first section provides an introduction to basic hemodynamic and angiocardiographic assessment, and a guide to some of the tools of the trade. The second section consists of specific case examples, discussing case planning, common techniques and pitfalls, results and outcomes. *It is important to note that the results discussed at the end of each case are specific to the practice of the institution where this manual originated.* Suggested further reading on other techniques and outcomes can be found at the end of the chapters; however, this is not an exhaustive list of available literature and largely represents a single institutional experience. The appendix includes useful charts and diagrams for reference.

Where credit is due
Finally, the early contributing authors to this manual were numerous, and many have long since progressed up the academic ladder to greater levels of fame and fortune. Regrettably, adequate credit and thanks cannot be given to all. It is the hope of those of us who have brought this manual to publication that the spirit of the original authors be carried forward in this and any subsequent revisions.

Known contributors and reviewers:

Laurie Armsby, MD	Doff McElhinney, MD
Charlie Baker, MD	Jeffery Meadows, MD
Lisa Bergersen, MD	Alan Nugent, MD
Susan Foerster, MD	Edward Rhee, MD
Steven Kamenir, MD	Ziad Saba, MD
Jackie Kreutzer, MD	Steven Seslar, MD
K.K. Kumar, MD	Nicole Sutton, MD
Michael Landzberg, MD	Rajiv Verma, MD
Barry Love, MD	Mark Warren, RN
Audrey C. Marshall, MD	

Special thanks:
   James Lock, MD
   Peter Lang, MD
   Stan Perry, MD
   Barry Keane, MD

–The Editors.

Part I
The Basics

Hemodynamics

When starting in the cath lab it is *essential* that you have an understanding of the findings as you collect them. This requires an understanding of normal intracardiac saturations and pressures (the only way to know when something is abnormal) and the calculations used for flow and resistance. All cardiologists must clearly understand not only the basis of the calculations, but also the limitations intrinsic to them.

In practice, most of the calculations for cardiac index, Qp:Qs, and pulmonary vascular resistance (PVR) can be estimated in one's head during the case as the saturations and pressures are being recorded. These estimates should then be compared to results generated by a computer, or more frequently by a calculator, later in the day after the examinations. If there is a large discrepancy, then it is likely the computer is wrong because you have selected incorrect data (e.g., Hematocrit put in as Hemoglobin).

Pressure Measurements

Accurate recording and interpretation of intracardiac pressure waveforms is paramount in a complete hemodynamic assessment. Before you record a pressure tracing you should be sure that it is of good quality and makes sense with what you know, or suspect, about the patient. It is, at best, a waste of time to record poor tracings. At their worst, poor tracings can lead to misinterpretation, inaccurate, or missed diagnoses.

Optimizing pressure waveforms for analysis requires some knowledge of the means by which they are transmitted and recorded. Complete understanding requires consideration of the sensitivity, natural frequency, and frequency response of the system. Fortunately, detailed reviews of pressure measurement systems can be found in standard cardiac catheterization textbooks. Hi-fidelity pressure catheters provide the most accurate tracings, but these can be quite expensive and fragile.

Practically speaking, most catheterization laboratory setups rely upon fluid-filled catheters for pressure transduction. These (and most types of systems) must be first "zeroed" to ambient air pressure. The standard reference point for this is the midpoint of the LA. With the transducer at this height, the transducer membrane is exposed to atmospheric pressure, and the monitor is then adjusted to zero. Then the monitoring system must be calibrated, a process that in most systems is performed automatically. Finally, if you are using more than one transducer, the transducers must be equilibrated. This is typically done by simultaneous pressure measurement at the same intracardiac/vascular location, or by measuring two pressures of similar magnitude, "switching ducers" to check that when the transducers are switched between catheters they indicate the same pressures.

When using a fluid filled catheter, a well-flushed (no air bubbles), large bore, stiff and short catheter will provide the most reliable waveforms. Of course, enthusiasm for a good waveform should be tempered by practical considerations of the patient's size and which catheters are needed for the procedure. Finally, remember, recognition of artifact is important. There are a host of artifacts that can mask or mimic pathophysiology.

L. Bergersen et al. (eds.), *Congenital Heart Disease*,
DOI 10.1007/978-0-387-77292-9_1, © Springer Science+Business Media, LLC 2009

Pressures and Waveforms

Right Atrial Pressure (RAp)

"Normal" right atrial pressure varies widely in response to myriad factors, including volume and respiratory status, heart rhythm, structure and function. "Normal" mean right atrial pressures for a child can be considered anywhere in the range 3–6 mmHg, although lower and occasionally negative values, particularly with inspiration or airway obstruction (snoring), are not infrequent. Many children with congenital heart disease (CHD) have elevated RAp, the long-term effects of which can be attested to by any physician caring for adults with CHD, Figure 1.

The normal right atrial pressure waveform consists of two, and sometimes three, positive waves (*a*, *c*, and *v*) followed by three negative deflections (*x*, *x'*, and *y*, respectively). The *a* wave results from atrial contraction (and is therefore absent in situations such as atrial fibrillation). Increased *a* waves are most frequently seen in situations of AV valve (AVV) stenosis, and AV dissociation when the atrium contracts against a closed AVV. Relatively increased *a* waves can occur with atrial contraction into noncompliant ventricles. The *x* decent follows the *a* wave and denotes atrial relaxation followed by AVV closure. The *c* wave is sometimes evident and occurs during ventricular systole as the closed AVV bulges into the atrium. While it is of physiologic interest, the clinical significance of the *c* wave is limited. The subsequent *x'* decent reflects the combined effects of continued atrial

relaxation and descent of the AVV during continued ventricular contraction. The *v* wave follows, denoting atrial filling while the AVV is still closed. The opening of the AVV followed by atrial emptying is represented by the *y* descent. The *y* descent is characteristically slowed in AVV stenosis. The subsequent period of slow or minimal ventricular filling with little change in atrial pressure (open AVV) is termed *diastasis* and is quickly followed by atrial contraction (*a* wave). RA pressures should drop with inspiration during spontaneous respiration, the absence of which is the hemodynamic equivalent of Kussmaul's sign.

Right Ventricular Pressure (RVp)

Normal (subpulmonary) right ventricular pressure also varies considerably with age, respiratory status, heart rhythm, structure, and function. Peak systolic pressure is typically 20–30 mmHg. End-diastolic pressure is typically equal or just slightly less than the right atrial *a* wave at 3–6 mmHg, Figure 2.

The right ventricular waveform is marked by a rapid rise during isovolumic contraction, followed by the peak systolic pressure before isovolumetric relaxation and a fall to minimum diastolic pressure (often near zero). There is a slow rise during diastolic filling during which a small RV "*a* wave" inflection may be seen as a result of atrial contraction just prior to end-diastole and subsequent isovolumic contraction.

This *a* wave, sometimes referred to as the *atrial kick*, frequently is accentuated in patients

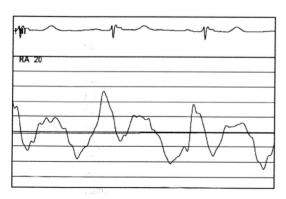

Fig. 1 Normal RA pressure waveform with a dominant A wave

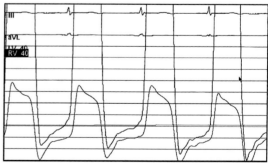

Fig. 2 Normal RV pressure waveform, simultaneous with LV pressure waveform

with first-degree AV bock. Peak RV systolic pressure is elevated in the presence of any downstream obstruction including right ventricular outflow obstruction (subPS or valvar PS), main or branch pulmonary artery stenosis, elevated pulmonary vascular resistance (pulmonary hypertension), or any lesion causing significant pulmonary venous or left atrial hypertension.

Pulmonary Artery Pressure (PAp)

The mean pulmonary artery pressure is usually less than 20 mmHg, with a systolic peak equal to or slightly less than that of the RVp, Figure 3. The pressure pulse is characterized by a relatively slow upstroke, peak systolic pressure, a small dicrotic notch, and slow fall to end diastole. The pulmonary artery pressure tracing provides in a single waveform significant insight into both right and left heart hemodynamics.

If you arrived at the PA through the right atrium and ventricle, a peak systolic pressure

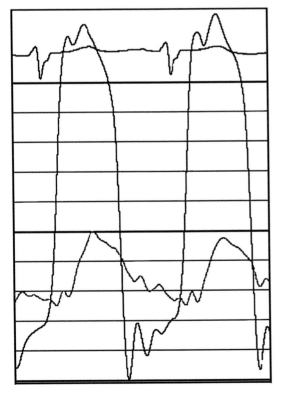

Fig. 3 Normal PA pressure waveform with simultaneous LV pressure waveform

significantly lower (>10 mmHg) than RV pressure denotes right ventricular outflow tract obstruction, which deserves further characterization to distinguish subvalvar, valvar, or supravalvar stenosis. Normally, there is a demonstrable diastolic pressure gradient between the PA and RV, the absence of which suggests truly "free" pulmonary regurgitation. Otherwise, the PA diastolic pressure more typically approaches the LA pressure.

Elevated PA pressures can occur with either increased flow (e.g., VSD), increased resistance (e.g., pulmonary vascular occlusive disease or PVOD), or downstream obstruction (e.g., left atrial hypertension). As such, it is important to use precise and unambiguous terminology. Remember that *pulmonary artery hypertension*, that is, high pulmonary artery pressure, is not synonymous with high pulmonary vascular resistance. For example, elevated PA pressures can occur with an unrestrictive VSD and normal pulmonary resistance. Full hemodynamic assessment is critical to distinguish between these, as important management decisions are based on the ability to manipulate the underlying process (e.g., you can replace/dilate a stenotic mitral valve, but you cannot as easily replace end-stage PVOD-affected lungs).

Pulmonary Capillary Wedge Pressure (PCWp)

A good pulmonary capillary wedge pressure (PCWp) resembles the left atrial pressure and waveform (Fig. 4) with a time delay of somewhere between 0.02 and 0.08 sec (Figure 4), unless there are significant collaterals or pulmonary vein stenosis. As such this waveform should have interpretable *a* and *v* waves and normal respiratory variation. An *underwedged* tracing usually has exaggerated systolic peaks as PAp is transmitted around the catheter. An *overwedged* PCWp typically lacks identifiable waveform morphology with a high drifting mean pressure.

Left Atrial Pressure (LAp)

In the normal heart, LA pressure is higher than RA pressure, with mean pressures in the range

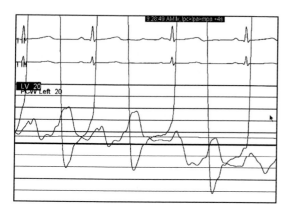

Fig. 4 Normal PCW$_P$ and LV waveform

Pulmonary Vein Wedge Pressure (PVWp)

The pulmonary venous wedge pressure (PVWp) operates under the same principle as the PCWp, but in the opposite direction, and provides a reasonable estimate of PAp (albeit often slightly underestimating), when the mean pressure obtained is less than 15 mmHg (above this, it is imprecise). When the PAp is a major reason for the catheterization and the patient is potentially unstable or access to the PAs may make them so, this can provide a quick estimate in case things go awry.

6–9 mmHg. Even with respiratory variation, LAp is never normally below atmospheric pressure.

The right and left atrial pressure waveforms are similar (Fig 5), but the *v* wave is usually dominant in the left atrium, ostensibly because of pulmonary venous contraction (e.g., the left atrial *a* wave is dominant in TAPVC). Increased *a* waves may be seen in mitral stenosis or in situations of poor LV compliance. Prosthetic mitral valves in the supra-annular position characteristically result in an increased *v* wave, probably due to the combined effects of a small, noncompliant LA and pulmonary venous contraction. However, increased *v* waves are more classically seen in mitral regurgitation. Overall, increased LAp can result from any of the above situations, significant left-to-right shunts, or LV dysfunction, Figure 5.

Left Ventricular Pressure (LVp)

The left ventricular pressure (LVp) varies with age and a host of structural and hemodynamic factors. Obviously, the peak systolic pressure should equal the ascending aortic pressure, failing which there must be is subvalvar, valvar, or supravalvar obstruction that warrants further characterization Figure 6. The LV end-diastolic pressure (LVEDp) is a crude but valuable marker for LV diastolic health, in that elevated LVEDp (>10–12 mmHg in children) suggests poor diastolic ventricular properties and/or LV failure. Similarly, a steep

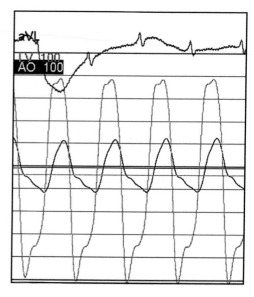

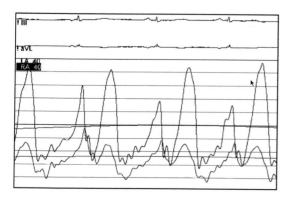

Fig. 5 Simultaneous RA and LA pressures

Fig. 6 LV and AO waveforms

slope of the diastolic portion of the LV waveform suggests poor ventricular compliance (see Figure 6 vs. Figure 4). "Normal" pressures vary according to age, with a progressive increase in the average LVEDp as patients progress to old age.

Aortic Pressure

The aortic pressure pulse varies uniquely in morphology in health and disease, much of which is due to timing and magnitude of reflected waves. Generally, there is systolic rise, peak aortic pressure, and a variable dicrotic notch on the downstroke Figure 6. A widened pulse pressure (systolic minus diastolic pressure) is characteristic of "run-off" lesions, including significant aortic (or neoaortic) regurgitation, PDA, surgical shunts or significant aorto-pulmonary collaterals. More commonly in adults than children, a widened pulse pressure may be seen in the setting of arterial stiffening and bradycardia. In contrast, a decreased or "narrow" pulse pressure may be seen in low cardiac output states and/or tamponade.

Pitfalls and Tips

As noted by Dr. Keane in the so-called "Green Book" (due to the color of its cover): "A catheterization is like a puzzle: everything must fit with everything else." If things do not fit, your case is probably not complete. The following are some tips about common problems:

- At the start of every case, ensure that you have a correct baseline and that the transducers are calibrated and equalized. This is easy to forget to do when things move fast. Remember that "re-zeroing" and re-equilibration between transducers may be required during the case.
- Know what to do with respiratory variation on a wave tracing. It is conventional to use the end-expiratory numbers, which are at the height of the tracing in spontaneously breathing patients and at the nadir in patients on positive pressure ventilation.
- Poor waveform morphology can result from either an *underdamped* or *overdamped* system.

Underdamped waveforms, demonstrated by *fling* or ringing, most commonly result from air in the catheter or transducer line, or the catheter position in a turbulent flow jet. The waveform has wide oscillation, high systolic spikes, and large negative overshoot waves. Try flushing the catheter or filling the catheter with blood or half-contrast. A similar appearance can occur with a catheter bouncing against the wall of the heart or vessel, in which case simple repositioning should work. The opposite, overdamped waveforms (sine wave), usually are the result of a loose connection or kinked catheter, and have a rounded out appearance with blunted and inaccurate limits. Checking the catheter and its connections or flushing the catheter will usually solve the problem.

- Remember to consider the patient's rhythm when you examine your waveforms. Nonsinus rhythm can drastically alter not only atrial waveform morphology but also absolute ventricular pressures and systolic flows.
- Finally, if the waveform you are getting does not make sense, consider that you may not be where you think you are in the heart, or your assumptions about the patient's physiology may be wrong. It is critically important to have the ability to rethink the patient's condition, and thereby the catheterization procedure, continuously throughout the case.

Assessment of Flows and Resistance

Calculated systemic and pulmonary flows (and their ratio) are important components of almost all catheterizations. The most common methods for obtaining these include calculations utilizing the methods originally conceived by Adolph Fick, and thermodilution (dye dilution being abandoned some time ago). Both of these have their assumptions and limitations that are important to remember.

The Fick Method

In 1870, Adolph Fick described a method for calculation of blood flow. He never tested his theory, but subsequent physiologists have, and the *Fick method* remains an important means of determining cardiac output. Indeed, the Fick method probably is the most common means by which cardiac flows are calculated in the pediatric catheterization lab.

Derivation of the equation is simple, and if the concept rather than equation is understood, the strengths and limitations of this method will never be forgotten. Stated simply, the total uptake (or release) of a substance by an organ is the product of blood flow to that organ and the concentration difference of the substance in the arteries and veins leading into and out of that organ. So, using arterial and venous oxygen content and oxygen consumption, one can easily calculate flow. Therefore, if oxygen content is:

Oxygen Content (mL O_2/dL plasma)

$= O_2$ bound to Hb + dissolved O_2

$= 1.36 \times$ Hgb $\times$ saturation $+ 0.003 \times PaO_2$

- 1.36 mL is the oxygen carrying capacity of 1 gm of hemoglobin.
- The relatively small amount of dissolved oxygen in plasma is 0.003 mL O_2/dL plasma/mmHg PaO_2.
- If the saturation is 98%, then use 0.98 in the formula, not 98.

then the important equation becomes:

Cardiac output (CO; L/min)

$$= \frac{O_2 \text{ consumption (mL } O_2/\text{min})}{AVO_2 \text{ content difference (\% mL } O_2/\text{dL)} \times 10}$$

* NOTE: Multiplication of the denominator by 10 is necessary to convert dL to L, if the hemoglobin is measured as g/dL.

Dissolved Oxygen

At 37°C, the solubility coefficient of O_2 is $\sim$0.003 mL O_2/dL plasma/mmHg PaO_2, or 0.3 ml O_2/dL plasma when PaO_2 is 100 mmHg. Normally, in room air, this represents approximately 1.5% of the total O_2 content and is usually ignored. If the patient is anemic, the proportion of dissolved O_2 increases. The addition of supplemental O_2 increases the contribution of the dissolved O_2 and must be included in calculations.

Oxygen Consumption (VO₂)

Oxygen consumption (VO_2) is often assumed, and is readily available in tables (see the appendix). There is variation based on sex, age, and heart rate. Unfortunately, studies comparing assumed and measured VO_2 show poor correlation and there are essentially no data published for the very small infant. Despite the limitations with assumed VO_2, this method remains widely used.

Oxygen consumption can be measured, using a hood. The process involves a gas pump that extracts all exhaled air and passes it through a mixing system and then measures oxygen content. The difference between inhaled oxygen content and exhaled oxygen content, with known flow by the pump, enables estimation of VO_2 (again based on the Fick principle). This assumes that no exhaled air is lost, that mixing is effective, and that volume of exhaled air equals volume of inhaled.

Common pitfalls and sources of inaccurate saturation measurements:

- Use of inappropriate or inaccurate mixed venous saturation.
- Samples not obtained as closely timed together as possible.
- Wedged instead of free PA sample with end-hole catheters (artificially high saturation).
- IVC saturations are inconsistent [both hepatic (low) and renal (high) are present].
- SVC saturation can be unusually high if there is reflux from ASD, PAPVR, arterio-venous malformations, or tricuspid regurgitation in the setting of a VSD.
- Failure to appreciate sedation-related hypoventilation during saturation assessment.
- Inappropriate pulmonary vein saturation assumption.
- Assumed oxygen consumption can be unreliable.
- If VO_2 is measured, inaccuracies can result if staff is unfamiliar with equipment.
- A catheter course mistaken for LA is actually coronary sinus (sat is usually 40–50%)
- Failure to include dissolved O_2 when in supplemental O_2.
- Small saturation differences can exist without a shunt (and vice versa).

Using these principles, both systemic and pulmonary flows can be calculated using the appropriate arterial and venous parameters. For pediatric catheterization, we most often express the indexed flow (to BSA), distinguishing between cardiac output (CO; L/min) and cardiac index (Qs; L/min/m^2). Because the VO$_2$ tables are usually indexed...

correction factors). This gives you a number which when divided by the relevant AVO$_2$ difference quickly gives you the indexed flow. For example:

An adult with a VO$_2$ of 125 ml/min/m^2 and a Hgb of 12.8gm/dl.

$$\text{Index systemic Flow (Qs)} = \frac{O_2 \text{ consumption (mL/min/}m^2)}{\text{Systemic arterial } O_2 \text{ content} - \text{Mixed venous } O_2 \text{ content}}$$

$$\text{Indexed pulmonary flow (Qp)} = \frac{O_2 \text{ consumption (mL/min/}m^2)}{\text{Pulmonary venous } O_2 \text{ content} - \text{Pulmonary arterial } O_2 \text{ content}}$$

Some general rules are the following:

- For mixed venous saturation with no shunts, use the PA saturation.
- If there is intracardiac shunting, use the SVC saturation for the mixed venous saturation. The SVC saturation used for calculations should never be higher than the PA saturation (unless there is anomalous pulmonary venous return or an oxygen-consuming tumor in the right ventricle!)
- If you do not directly obtain a pulmonary vein or LA saturation, assume something appropriate to the clinical status of the patient, ~95–100% in the absence of lung disease.
- In practice, when a patient is breathing room air (~21% FiO$_2$) we neglect the relatively small contribution of dissolved oxygen to the oxygen content. This greatly simplifies the math, but should *not* be done when the patient is receiving supplemental oxygen.
- Always document all assumptions in your catheterization report.

- Make sure your numbers make sense.

Tip: The Hgb and the oxygen-carrying capacity of Hgb (the 1.36) are essentially the same in both the arterial and venous samples. If you do not have to include dissolved oxygen you can make approximate calculations during the case easier by doing half the math ahead of time. One way is the following: Divide the VO$_2$ by the product of the Hgb and 0.136 (includes

Your predetermined "number" derived as described above is 125/(12.8*0.136) = 72. If the MVO$_2$ saturation is 79% and the aortic saturation is 99%, then 72/(99 – 79) = ~3.6 L/min/m^2. Always double check and confirm your math.

Qp:Qs Calculation

In patients with structural heart disease, mixing is common (and often necessary), making important the concept of the ratio of pulmonary to systemic blood flow (also known as Qp:Qs). Conveniently, much of the above formulae cancel out, leaving a simple equation:

$$\text{Qp:Qs} = \frac{\text{Ao sat} - \text{MV sat}}{\text{PV sat} - \text{PA sat}}$$

For example, take a situation where the only structural problem is an atrial septal (ASD), as shown in Figure 7. In performing a hemodynamic run you find an SVC (mixed venous) saturation of 75% with PA saturations of 84% and equal pulmonary vein and aortic saturations of 99%. The net Qp:Qs in this patient is (99 – 75)/(99 – 84) = 1.6.

Now consider a patient with hypoplastic left heart syndrome (HLHS) with shunt physiology Figure 8.

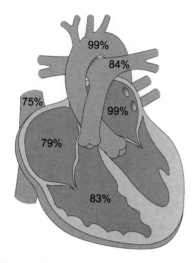

Fig. 7 ASD with saturation measurements

Table 1. Variation in Qp:Qs with shunted single ventricle physiology

	Qp:Qs	Arterial saturation (%)
MV sat 50%	0.5	67
	1	75
	2	83
	3	88
MV sat 70%	0.5	80
	1	85
	2	90

(a pulmonary venous saturation of 100% has been assumed).

In this patient you only need to know the SVC, pulmonary vein (sometimes assumed) and aortic saturations in order to calculate the net Qp:Qs because the only source of pulmonary blood flow is the shunt; therefore, the pulmonary artery saturation is equal to the aortic saturation. So, with an SVC saturation of 69%, pulmonary vein saturations of 99% and an aortic saturation of 87%, the net Qp:Qs is ~1.7. This is a similar net Qp:Qs as the ASD above but obviously the physiology is completely different. To give you an idea of how changes in mixed venous and arterial saturations affect Qp:Qs in a patient with this kind of shunted physiology consider Table 1

Thermodilution

First introduced in the 1950s, the principle of thermodilution involves determining the extent and rate of thermal changes in the blood stream related to injection of a fixed volume of fluid at a set temperature upstream. From this temperature–time curve and knowledge of the magnitude of the initial heat change, the volume rate of flow can be calculated in a manner analogous to that used for dye and other indicator–dilution methods. The decision to use thermodilution versus Fick depends on your needs and your staff interventionalist's preference.

Technique

A thermodilution catheter is placed with the tip resting free in the PA and the proximal port in the RA. If the patient is <15 kg we generally use a 5 Fr catheter (5-cc syringe) and if the patient is >15 kg we generally use a 7 Fr catheter (10-cc syringe). After an exact amount of solution (either room temperature or iced) is injected through a side lumen in the RA, the change in temperature is sensed by a thermistor located at the tip of the catheter. Always check to be sure that you are infusing the *proximal* port (yes, it has happened). The first syringe serves to cool down the catheter shaft and is usually ignored. The next three samples are averaged. The three recordings should be within 15–20% of each other, that is, it is normal to have some scatter.

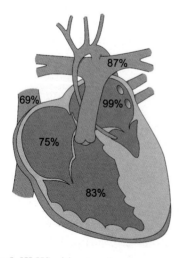

Fig. 8 HLHS with saturation measurements

Don't forget to index the output. This technique is most often used in aortic valve, mitral valve, and coarctation dilations, and occasionally in ICU patients.

Common Problems

- High cardiac output will cause only a small temperature drop, increasing the risk for error.
- If the thermistor tip lies on or near the PA wall (the wall serves as heat sink) this can produce a falsely high output.
- If the proximal port is not in free flowing blood, there will be loss of temperature before reaching the thermistor.
- Respiration causes a small change in PA temperature (negligible).
- Slow injection of cooled solution will produce a smaller magnitude temperature change, falsely elevating the calculated cardiac output.
- If the incorrect catheter size is put into the computer, the output may be incorrect, that is, if using a 5 Fr catheter but 7 Fr is entered into the computer, then the CO will be falsely elevated ($2 \times$ CO). Similar errors will occur if you use the wrong syringe (5 cc or 10 cc). Similarly, the temperature of the injectate must be known and properly entered.

Resistance Calculations

The concept (and reality) of resistance to blood flow is important in patients being considered for many surgical interventions. Using the results of your flow calculations above and your pressure measurements, you can assess resistance. Doing so involves a simple variation on Ohm's law where $R = V/I$ becomes

$$\text{Resistance} = \Delta \text{Pressure/Flow}$$

Therefore, PVR (pulmonary vascular resistance) or total pulmonary resistance is given as

$$(\text{PVR}) = \frac{\text{meanPAp} - \text{meanLAp}}{\text{Qp}}$$

- PVR is usually indexed and expressed as indexed Wood units (mmHg/L/min/m^2).
- Normal PVR is <2 indexed Wood units (WU)
- If you are talking to an adult cardiologist they may be more familiar with resistance expressed in the metric units of dynes/sec $\times$ cm^{-5}. Multiply WU $\times$ 80 for conversion, and note if the number is indexed.
- Make sure that when you assess resistance you check the pH and pCO_2, to exclude iatrogenic pulmonary vasoconstriction and falsely elevated PVR.

Using the same principles, systemic vascular resistance is...

$$\text{SVR} = \frac{\text{mean Aop} - \text{mean RAp}}{\text{Qs (indexed)}}$$

- Normal SVR 15 – 20 WU.

Nitric Trials

The rationale for testing pulmonary vasoreactivity is based upon the predictive utility of "responders" to NO in responding to other agents. The catheterization procedure is relatively straight forward.

1. Test baseline flows, Qp:Qs (when relevant) and PVR.
2. After 10 minutes of 100% O_2, remeasure everything, and calculate PVR (remember to include dissolved O_2!).
3. After 10 minutes of 100% O_2 and nitric oxide 20–80 ppm (we usually do this once at 80 ppm), do it again.

Assessment of PVR is particularly important in the following patient groups:

- Prior to partial and complete cavopulmonary anastomoses (Glenn/Fontan) in single ventricle patients, because the risk of postoperative complications increases in patients with PVR > 3WU.
- For risk stratification in patients prior to transplant, as the risk of postoperative right heart failure is higher in patients with a PVR > 6WU, even in the presence of O2 or NO.

- To assess vascular responsiveness in patients with pulmonary hypertension related to increased PVR, which can predict responsiveness to medical therapies for these patients.

Constriction, Restriction, and Effusion

The physiologic changes that accompany these disease processes have long been of clinical and intellectual interest to cardiologists. The following are general characteristics of each. Remember that there is some overlap with these findings, and sensitivity can be lacking. Therefore, appropriate evaluation and conclusions require a complete knowledge of the clinical scenario. Because effusions are usually easily demonstrable by echocardiography, the usual difficulty arises from distinguishing restriction (myocardial disease) from constriction (pericardial disease).

Constrictive Pericardial Disease

While this is a relatively uncommon process in pediatric cardiology, it may be more common in adults with CHD, and it remains an important consideration in any patient with unexplained diastolic dysfunction.

Classic findings include elevation and equalization (within 5 mmHg) of right and left atrial and ventricular end-diastolic pressures. There may be loss of the normal RAp decline with inspiration (Kussmaul's sign). RA waveforms demonstrate a preserved x and prominent y descent, often with equal a and v waves, giving the classic appearance of the "M" or "W" sign. Both RV and LV pressure waveforms demonstrate an early and prominent diastolic "dip" and rapid rise to a "plateau" resulting in the classic "dip and plateau," or "square root" sign.

In patients with tachycardia this sign may be difficult to appreciate. In such cases, the prolonged diastole that follows an induced PVC will occasionally unmask this phenomena. RV end diastolic pressure is frequently $> 1/3$ RV systolic pressure, but RV and PA systolic pressures are usually only moderately elevated. Relative hypovolemia can rarely mask some of these

findings but may be elicited by rapid infusion of volume. The sensitivity of these findings is quite high (90–95%) but the positive and negative predictive values range widely, from 4–92%.

Characteristic respiratory variations (during spontaneous respiration) may provide the most sensitive and specific criteria for constrictive disease and may be of particular use in distinguishing constrictive from restrictive disease. The first of these is the finding of ventricular discordance, or *ventricular interdependence*, manifest by an inspiratory increase in systolic RVp with simultaneous decrease in systolic LVp (in contrast to the normal state where RV and LVp rise and fall together). Also, it has been suggested that in constrictive pericardial disease, normal changes in intrathoracic pressure are prevented from being fully transmitted to the intracardiac structures. As such, there is a decrease in the early diastolic transmitral gradient (LA or PCWp minus minimum LV early diastolic pressure) with inspiration, whereas normally there is no change. The latter finding may be subtle and may require the use of hi-fidelity catheters to be appreciated, but the former finding is reported to have positive and negative predictive values in the 95–100% range.

Restrictive Disease

Hemodynamic findings in restrictive disease can mimic those of chronic constrictive disease. The "M" sign and Kussmaul's sign may be seen, but atrial pressures tend to be higher than those observed with constrictive disease. Likewise, the "dip and plateau" sign may occasionally be seen with restriction, although LV diastolic pressures tend to remain higher than those of the RV (lack of equalization). Secondary pulmonary hypertension is more common in restriction than constriction, and therefore RV and PA systolic pressures can be higher.

Effusive Pericardial Disease (and Tamponade)

We do not usually evaluate intracardiac hemodynamics in patients with isolated pericardial effusions. However, occasionally you will have reason to catheterize a patient who happens to have some degree of pericardial fluid and you will need to know its significance. Perhaps more importantly, you will need to promptly recognize the hemodynamic alterations that signify unrecognized heart perforation during a case leading to progressive tamponade. In these cases the following points are important to consider.

High pericardial pressure exerts its primary hemodynamic effect by impeding right heart filling. There is equalization of atrial and ventricular end-diastolic pressures; closest during inspiration (during spontaneous respiration) and a gross reduction in intracardiac volumes (both end-diastolic and end-systolic volumes are reduced). With respect to the RA waveform (and jugular venous pressure) classically there is loss of the y descent (poor early diastolic filling), attributed to a fixed intracardiac volume. *Pulsus paradoxus* may be observed in aortic pressure tracings, with a greater than 10 mmHg systolic pressure decline with inspiration. Of note, close attention to a pulse oximetry tracing may show exaggerated respiratory variation as well.

Fortunately, in contrast to restrictive and constrictive disease, effusive disease with tamponade is acutely remediable, although in rare cases relief of tamponade can reveal underlying restrictive or constrictive disease.

Additional Readings

Grossman W. Section III: hemodynamic principles (pp. 131–184). In: *Grossman's Cardiac Catheterization, Angiography, and Intervention*. Donald S. Baim (ed.). 7th ed. Lippincott Williams & Wilkins, Philadelphia PA, 2006.

Keane JF, Lock JE. Hemodynamic evaluation of congenital heart disease (pp. 37–72). In: *Diagnostic and Interventional Catheterization in Congenital Heart Disease*, 2 nd ed. Kluwer Academic Publishers, Norwell, MA, 2000.

Kern M. *Hemodynamic Rounds*. 2 nd ed. Wiley-Liss. New York, 1999.

Yang SS, Bentivoglio Y, Maranhao V et al. *From Cardiac Catheterization Data to Hemodynamic Parameters*. 3rd ed. F.A. Davis Company, hiladelphia. 1978.

NOTE: Waveforms were copied from cases performed at Children's Hospital Boston.

Precatheterization Assessment and Preparation

Cardiac catheterization in the patient with congenital heart disease shares few common elements with routine cardiac catheterization in the adult with isolated coronary or even valvular heart disease. Indeed, although many of the tools are similar, the indications for catheterization, the techniques used, and interventions performed are widely diverse. Nevertheless, both types of procedures require careful preparation that is individualized to the specific patient and case.

The distillation of all your careful preparation and planning is the "workup," which you will be called upon to do for your own cases, and occasionally for others. The essential steps of this process include:

1. Obtain a focused history. Learn and know well the initial cardiac anatomy. Know not just *what* surgeries the patient has had performed but *how* and by *whom* they were done. There are numerous and important variations on even the simplest surgery and many have bearing on what you will do in the lab. Know the access sites, hemodynamic measurements, and interventions performed at prior catheterizations. Know the current clinical status of the patient and the reason for the present catheterization. Think about other medical problems and how they affect your case (e.g., renal insufficiency or airway management issues).
2. Obtain informed consent (see section on obtaining consent).
3. Examine the patient. Look for signs and symptoms associated with their diagnosis. **Know** their pulses, and look for signs of venous occlusion (e.g., prominent superficial vessels, etc.)
4. Review the data. A good catheterization scheduling sheet should include room for the referring physician to request appropriate preprocedural studies (e.g., CXR, lung scan, echo, etc.). When you review this sheet, make sure the patient needs these studies, decide (before the patient goes home if they have come in the prior day) if they need any additional studies (pre- *or* postcatheterization) and make sure they all get done or scheduled, and then review the studies for any surprises.
5. Plan the case (see section on planning the case)
6. Plan for after the case. Think about what the patient will need postcatheterization. Note that it is often difficult to obtain certain studies (e.g., lung scans) on a weekend. If you have a Friday case that needs a lung scan or echo afterwards, discuss this with your attending physician early. The follow-up study can often be done at a later date. If not, consider getting the study on the way to the floor after the case, or call the department performing the test and plead to have it done the following day. If special medications are needed, try to arrange for them ahead of time. Anticipate who may need the ICU after catheterization and let the charge nurse know of the possibility prior to the case.

Obtaining Consent

This is a routine task. You will do it hundreds of times; you may even develop a canned speech for most cases; but **this is important**. In most cases, the faculty catheterizer or the patient's primary cardiologist will have already explained the case to the patient or parent. Your job is to be sure they really understand.

L. Bergersen et al. (eds.), *Congenital Heart Disease*,
DOI 10.1007/978-0-387-77292-9_2, © Springer Science+Business Media, LlC 2009

Explain the Procedure

Make sure the patient knows what you plan to do, and why. If this is his or her first catheterization, they may not know anything, so be patient and thoughtful. If this is their 30th case, they may not be listening. Be sure they are. Every case is different. Discuss *anything* that could be done, even if you think it is unlikely. Tell the patient that you may not do what you had planned if the information you obtain during the procedure suggests a change in management. Also discuss the possibility that success may be incomplete (residual device leak) or that you may fail in your efforts. It does happen. Make sure the location of the parents is known during the catheterization in case permission is needed for some unexpected reason.

Discuss All Potential Complications

Pain, bleeding with the potential need for blood transfusion, infection, allergic reaction, blood vessel or heart damage or even perforation, arrhythmia, heart block, hemodynamic instability with resulting end organ damage (kidney, brain, etc.), seizure, stroke, and death—these can all happen, even in simple hemodynamic procedures. Remember, serious morbidity and mortality can result from central venous or arterial cannulation, and this is the first and often simplest thing you will do. Do not be so sure that complications will not happen to *your* patient.

If a valvotomy is anticipated, then add damage to the valve causing regurgitation with a need for surgical repair or replacement.

If a coil or stent is being placed, then add embolization with the possibility of causing injury to other organs or occlusion of unintended vessels requiring removal by trans-catheter methods or surgery.

If a septal or vascular occlusion device is going to be placed, then add device malposition or embolization requiring removal in the catheterization lab or by surgery. Also explain any cardiac or extracardiac structures that could be damaged by an embolized device. Know the device that is likely to be used and the complications more likely to occur with that device. Discuss the possibility of development of thrombus on the device.

Planning the Case

You would not jump out of an airplane without a parachute. Similarly, you should not enter the catheterization lab unless you have a plan and also a back-up plan for your patient. When planning your case, the first question you need to ask is, "Why, exactly, are we doing this catheterization?" The answer to this question will guide your planning of and decision-making during the case, and (importantly) will help you to decide when you have completed your case. During your first month in the catheterization laboratory you should (and are encouraged to) ask senior fellows for assistance in planning your cases. They will advise you on important details.

There is much to think about in planning a case. At a minimum, you should consider and plan for the following:

Sedation

- Is PO or IV nursing sedation appropriate for the case, or should the cardiac anesthesia staff be consulted?
- If you think general anesthesia is required, consider its consequences in terms of obtaining hemodynamics, case scheduling, and postcatheterization care.
- See "More on Sedation Planning" below.

Access

- Which vessels? Based on where you need to go and the history of vascular occlusion.
- What size sheaths? Determined by which pictures you want and what size catheters you need to perform intended measurements/interventions.

Hemodynamic Data:

- Where do you want to obtain saturations and pressures? How will you obtain these data?
- What is the relative priority of the pieces of hemodynamic data?

- What do you expect to find?
- What do you not expect to find but need to prove?

Calculations

- What numbers do you need to calculate CI, PVR, Qp/Qs?
- If you are not measuring it, what is the patient's assumed VO_2?
- What is the patient's hemoglobin?
- How and when will you calculate these values during the case?
- Can you use standard equations with the patient's physiology?

Angiography

- What pictures do you want to take, how should they be prioritized?
- How much contrast and how quickly should it be delivered?
- What size and type of catheter will accommodate the volume and rate of contrast?
- What camera angles will you need to take a good angiogram?
- What is the patient's renal status?

Interventions

- What interventions are you planning, or are possible for your case?
- How will you determine if an intervention is indicated?
- What criteria are used to pick an appropriate-sized device, coil, or balloon?
- What are the potential complications of a given procedure?
- How does one intervention affect another and in what sequence will you do them?

Disposition

- What studies or medications will your patient need following the catheterization?
- Will the patient be discharged to home or be admitted to the cardiology ward?
- Is the child likely to become ill during or following the catheterization and need an ICU bed?

More on Sedation Planning

Deciding on the type of sedation for your case requires knowledge of the patient's cardiac and noncardiac medical history, the patient's history of prior sedations and medication reactions, practical considerations about access and additional procedures, and finally, the type of procedure you have planned.

Cardiac Considerations

This should include how sick the patient is presently and how sick they are likely to become during the catheterization. By now, you know that "sickness" can manifest in many ways, but always start by considering the patient's myocardial function and reserve. Children with very poor function may not tolerate even the slightest bit of sedation, associated hypoventilation, or hypotension. Consider your expected interventions.

Balloon dilation (causing complete obstruction) of ventricular outflow without a "pop-off" (PFO, ASD, VSD) is tolerated differently under different physiologic states. Also consider your patients' propensity for arrhythmia and how well they are likely to tolerate it. Finally, don't forget the lungs! Their physiologic relation to the heart (in the middle or before) makes them susceptible to downstream sequelae of your interventions (e.g., reperfusion edema and hemorrhage in TOF/PA with multiple PA dilations, or obstructive pulmonary edema with pulmonary vein or mitral valve dilations).

Noncardiac Considerations

Just because it's "not the heart" doesn't mean that it isn't important. Remember to consider noncardiac medical problems, including: airway abnormalities, pulmonary disease (asthma, BPD, single lungs, etc.), reflux, hepatic, genetic issues (Trisomy 21) and renal failure (drug metabolism). In sick infants, just having the hips elevated for access (see part on access) can cause considerable respiratory compromise from diaphragm elevation and shifting of abdominal contents.

Sedation History

Prior sedation history plays a key role in how you plan sedation for your procedure. A child with multiple failed sedations is likely to do the same unless they have aged several years, etc. Further, infants and children who have seen a great deal of medications in their recent history due to surgery or hospitalization are likely to require higher doses or alternative sedation strategies. Remember to ask about allergies and paradoxical reactions to your usual armamentarium, and also look for a history of malignant hyperthermia.

Practical Considerations

Access in places such as the neck, shoulder, or liver can be *distressing* to a conscious child or even adult. These access routes are also often technically more difficult, requiring better sedation and immobilization. Finally, if you are going to need another procedure (e.g., TEE, bronchoscopy) you are probably going to need general anesthesia. In sick older patients, if they cannot lie flat in bed (due to ascites or congestive heart failure) without sedation, then it is very unlikely that they will tolerate sedation without considerable decompensation.

Despite these many considerations, your decision tree with respect to arranging sedation for your case is relatively simple.

1. Who is going to do the sedation?
   Option 1: You and the nurse.
   Option 2: The anesthesiologist (general or cardiac).
   Option 3: CICU staff (this is rare, usually only if the patient is coming from the CICU and no anesthesiologist is available).
2. How much sedation does the patient need?
   Option 1: Conscious sedation (which is best when baseline cardiorespiratory assessments are important, e.g., pulmonary HTN and vasodilator testing).
   Option 2: General anesthesia with intubation.
   Option 3: Various advanced nongeneral anesthesia options per anesthesia.

In many institutions, an anesthesiologist is a sparse resource. Everyone's life will be easier if you remember that in most institutions there are a finite number of staff anesthesiologists available. They cannot possibly staff all the operating rooms, the rest of the hospital, and all the catheterization labs at the same time. Consider this and remember that it may dictate the order of your cases. A good catheterization scheduling sheet should have some kind of a check box if anesthesia is requested. If it is not clear during your workup why anesthesia is needed, either you do not have all the information, or the patient may not really need anesthesia involvement. Talk with your attending physician and/or the referring cardiologist and make a decision early. Alternatively, you may decide that a patient not scheduled for anesthesia should have it. Again, discuss this with the relevant staff.

Scheduling Cases

Case scheduling varies from institution to institution. If you are given some part in this process, don't consider yourself blessed. Scheduling cases can be more of an art than a science and some days there will be no good solution that will satisfy all involved. Here are some general points to remember when making a schedule. These guidelines will be broken many times but they will provide a framework of how to assemble a schedule.

1. In institutions with multiple catheterization labs, often some rooms have different imaging and support capabilities. If you are doing a "hybrid" case, do not schedule the case in a room without support for this.
2. Schedule outpatients earlier in the day than inpatients or patients scheduled for admission postcatheterization. Anyone with the potential to go home (e.g., PDA or hemodynamics) after their catheterization should usually go first.
3. Younger kids should precede older kids. It is usually harder to keep toddlers and young children NPO all morning.
4. Try to keep all of a given attending physician's catheterization cases in the same room. (This may result in violation of rule 1.)

5. As mentioned above, anesthesia is often short-staffed and can be the limiting factor in scheduling cases. Talk with them early and stagger anesthesia cases if necessary. If you have any questions ask a senior fellow.
6. It is a good idea to schedule very complex cases first, if possible, when the staff's energy level is high!
7. All of the above rules can and should be violated if a critically ill patient requires catheterization.

Case Presentation

Precatheterization case conference is an important part of the precatheterization process. At many institutions this occurs each morning before the cases begin, and it is here that all the cases for the day are discussed. At other institutions this may be a simple one-on-one discussion with the fellow and attending physician. Either way, by this point you should have prepared for and planned out your case in detail. Here is when you get to lay out your plan. Your case presentation should be brief, but you should know any and all relevant details if asked.

Bring or have available the following items for your presentation:

- Catheterization report(s) and angiograms.
- Chest X-ray.
- Lung scan results and image.
- EKG.
- Most recent echocardiogram report and images.
- Operative report(s).

The presentation should include the patient's past cardiac medical, surgical, and catheterization history. The prior catheterization history should mention occlusion of vessels, and pertinent hemodynamic data and interventions with knowledge of size of devices or balloons used. If stents had been placed previously you should note the largest balloon used to dilate the stent. If sites were difficult to access, the successful catheter or technique should be discussed. Vital signs and physical exam findings should be presented including the height and weight, physical findings, and presence of pulses. The CXR and EKG should be presented followed by the echocardiogram and the angiograms. (Be sure that you have reviewed these before conference.) Following the patient presentation you should present your plan for the case and any questions you may have.

In the Lab

In contrast to cardiac catheterization in adults, cases in patients with structural heart disease are seldom predictable. Even the most routine catheterization in a patient with congenital heart disease can reveal unexpected findings that completely change the expected course of the procedure. With that said, most cases start and proceed in logical sequence. All cases begin with setting up the table and getting access. Hemodynamic assessment is next, usually followed by angiography and, finally, intervention, if warranted. This is the usual sequence, although exceptions do exist.

Setting-Up the Table

Every case starts with preparing the table. This is where all your equipment is initially placed and prepared for use during the case. The contents of the table will vary from institution but usually include the following at a minimum:

- Gowns, drapes and towels (to cover the patient and physician).
- Syringes and needles of many sizes (for obvious and not-so-obvious purposes).
- A basin for sharps and waste.
- Transducers.
- In-line "closed system" for saline and contrast.
- CO_2 system (essentially a stopcock and a length of tubing).
- Your selected sheaths, catheters, and wires.
- Miscellaneous: sterile covers for imaging equipment, handle for overhead light, etc.

The actual process of setting up the table varies from person to person, and a more senior fellow should be present to help you the first couple of times. Occasionally you will have the good fortune of having the laboratory technicians or support staff set it up for you. But at the start, you should learn to set up the table yourself Fig. 1. The whole process should take less than 5 minutes when you have the hang of it. In the beginning, give yourself more time. Don't delay the case because you are still setting up the table. The following are a few final tips.

- Set up the basins and syringes early so the techs can fill the basins with saline and the cup with contrast.
- Obtain your heparin and lidocaine early and give the lidocaine to the patient sooner rather then later, because it takes time (at least 5 minutes) to reach full effect.
- Ask for bicarb for your lidocaine to decrease injection pain (admittedly, studies on efficacy are mixed).
- Do not stick the technician with the needle when getting the lidocaine.
- Drape the patient as soon as you can. The attending can walk in at any time and may want to start getting access while you finish setting up the table (or vice versa).

Vascular Access

General Considerations

There are two rules you need to remember about access:

Rule #1: You can't cath if you don't have access.

Rule #2: When you have access, don't lose it!

L. Bergersen et al. (eds.), *Congenital Heart Disease*,
DOI 10.1007/978-0-387-77292-9_3, © Springer Science+Business Media, LLC 2009

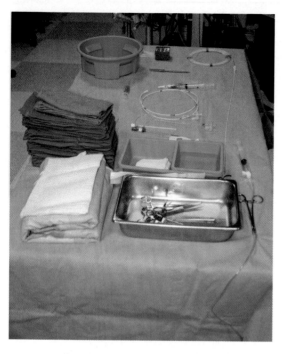

Fig. 1 Equipment table

Some questions you need to ask yourself to help decide on vascular access are:

- *Where has the patient been accessed previously?* For example, if a patient has had multiple caths, has recent access been from the left femoral vein? If so, it may be because the right is occluded.
- *Are there vessels that are documented to be occluded by angiography, or is occlusion surmised because of a failed attempt?* Check previous cath reports and look at the old angios.
- *Where do I need to go?* For example, if cathing a patient with a bidirectional Glenn, you cannot usually get to the pulmonary arteries from the femoral vein.
- *What access will make the procedure I am doing the easiest?* For example, for a Brockenbrough puncture, access from the RFV is generally easier than the LFV.
- *Are there lines already in place?* Can these lines be used for the case, and what is currently infusing through them?
- *Do I need to leave the lines in post-cath?* Access "from above" (subclavian or internal jugular vein) is better in anyone but a baby if

you plan on leaving lines in for care in the ICU. Umbilical lines are sometimes useful to leave in for post-cath care in the newborn.

Keeping the above points in mind, before you get access you need to know how you are going to maintain it. You have essentially two options. First, you can simply leave a catheter in the blood vessel, or second, you can place a sheath. A sheath is a tapered catheter (usually with a hemostasis valve and side-port for flushing) that stays in the vessel and permits catheter changes and exchanges without constantly passing a catheter across the arteriotomy or venotomy (i.e., causing vessel damage). All sheaths come with a removable tapered dilator that fits closely around a specified wire and minimizes vessel and soft tissue trauma as the sheath is placed. The nominal French size of the sheath is the size of the largest catheter that can fit through the lumen of the sheath. So, if you are planning to use a 7-Fr wedge catheter, you'll need at least a 7-Fr sheath (which is closer to 8 Fr in external diameter).

Venous Access

Because multiple catheter manipulations and changes are often required in the venous system we routinely use a sheath in the vein. The size (diameter) of the sheath depends on the size of the catheter you need to put through it. In general, start with the size of the catheter with which you plan to do hemodynamics and angiography, and then if a larger sheath is needed for interventions you can upsize as needed. If you are pretty sure you will need a larger sheath later, you may also consider starting with it. Otherwise, because the most common balloon endhole catheters are 5 Fr and 7 Fr this can guide your initial sheath selection. For example, if you plan on using a balloon end-hole catheter for hemodynamics, choose a 5 Fr for an infant or child (<15–20 Kg) and 7 Fr for a larger child or adult. A 4 Fr sheath also may be considered in a very small child, but recognize that this may limit your subsequent catheter choices somewhat.

If you are using a thermodilution catheter for hemodynamics, remember that there are four lumens in these catheters (end hole, side hole, balloon, and thermister) and only a really tiny (~useless) wire will generally fit through the end hole. In addition, because there are two lumens for the same French size, the lumens are small and do not transduce pressures well. Therefore, only use the 5 Fr thermodilution catheter in infants and small children <15 kg; otherwise you probably will prefer the 7 Fr thermodilution catheter.

The other consideration in choosing a sheath is the length. We almost always start with a short sheath. The actual length of the "short" sheath varies with the Fr size. The sheaths are intended to reach the common iliac vein from the access site. So, for example, a 5 Fr sheath typically used for a newborn cath needs to be only 7.5 cm long, whereas an 8 Fr sheath in an obese adolescent will likely need to be 11 cm long. Short sheaths are available in sizes 3 Fr to >20 Fr, in increments of one Fr size up to a 12 Fr, and then in increments of two Fr sizes beyond that (e.g., 12, 14, etc.). All short sheaths have an integral hemostasis valve and sidearm. Long sheaths come in a variety of lengths, shapes, and characteristics. The most common long sheaths vary from 45 to 90 cm in length. Not all long sheaths have an integral hemostasis valve and sidearm so you may need to place one yourself. Long sheaths are most often used for the placement of stents and devices, or to secure distal access during PA dilation cases.

Arterial Access

The most common site for arterial access is the femoral arteries, although umbilical and radial are also used. For femoral arterial access, a sheath is not always necessary. If you only want to measure pressures and take angiograms with a single catheter (usually a pigtail) you can simply place that catheter over your access wire and use that for your case. In contrast, if you anticipate multiple catheter manipulations or exchanges you should probably place an arterial sheath. Either way, the most common starting arterial catheter (sheath or no sheath) is a pigtail catheter.

The two variables that determine the size of the pigtail catheter you need are:

1. The amount and rate of contrast needed for angiography, and
2. The patient's length (the pigtail must be ~ 2/3 of the patient length to reach the apex of the ventricle in a patient with a left aortic arch, and slightly longer if there is a right aortic arch).

Consult the Appendix in this book to help determine the size of pigtail you need. If you just need arterial access for monitoring, a short pigtail of small diameter will do. If you are using a pigtail catheter without a sheath and you get access with a 0.018″ torque wire, be aware that the wire-catheter lumen mismatch can cause arterial trauma as you advance your catheter. Alternatively, if you want to monitor blood pressure during prolonged left-sided interventions, choosing a sheath size that is one to two Fr sizes larger than your catheters will allow you to transduce arterial pressure throughout the case through the side-arm of the sheath.

Technique

The techniques of access described here are all based upon the modified Seldinger technique, which obtains vascular access using a catheter over-a-wire. Seldinger first described this technique in 1953 but it took a while to catch on. Until the early 1970s, access was obtained primarily with a cut-down (surgical) technique. Now that we are proficient at the Seldinger technique, a cutdown is almost never required.

Tools of the Trade

Before you start attempting to get access you should familiarize yourself with the needles and wires commonly used in the catheterization lab, because they are different from those you are probably used to.

Needles

First you need to choose the right needle for access. Generally, we use Cook® access needles. They come in a variety of sizes, which are all color-coded. The most popular sizes are the "pink" ones (18 gauge), which accept a 0.035″

wire (needed for some 5 Fr–6 Fr and all larger sheaths), and the "brown" ones (19 gauge) which accept a 0.025″ (19 gauge) wire or 0.035″ gauge. "Yellow" ones are 20 gauge and accept a 0.018″ wire. If you use these, remember to use as short of a needle as possible, because the resistance from the small lumen can be greater than the venous pressure in longer needles—or more plainly, you may not see a "flash."

"Green" (21 gauge) needles usually come in a Micropuncture® perc kit that includes a short floppy 0.018″ torque, with an inner dilator which follows the 0.018″ wire and larger outer dilator. After the wire position is secured, the inner dilator may be removed and 0.018″ wire, leaving an outer dilator that accepts an 0.035″ wire compatible with 7 F sheaths. These kits are useful when you are placing a 7 F sheath but want to use a smaller needle. After the vessel is accessed, place the combination dilator over the wire. The inner dilator is then removed with the 0.018″ wire and a 0.035″ wire is placed. The outer dilator is then removed over this wire and the 7 F sheath is placed.

Usually, because many patients with structural heart disease have elevated central venous pressure, we perc with just the needle, with no syringe on the back. If you are attempting access with a syringe on the back of the needle (e.g., for an IJV) there is often no reason to use a larger needle, because you are probably already applying gentle suction. In these situations we often prefer the yellow or green needle for insertion of smaller sheaths.

All of the access needles described here have a bevel that makes them sharp. One problem with these needles is that they will give blood return even if only part of the needle lumen is in the vessel. This is particularly true for needles with long bevels. If a wire is advanced in this situation, it may not enter the vessel without repositioning. Additionally, most needles are sharpened along the distal beveled sides, so side-to-side manipulation of the needle can result in laceration of tissue or vessels. Be aware of both of these properties as you use the needles.

Wires

A more detailed description of wires is given latter in this manual, but you should be familiar

with those commonly employed in obtaining access. Your options are to use the wires that come with the sheaths (if you are using a sheath), or to use more fancy (expensive) wires. The advantage of wires that come with the sheaths is that you know they work with those sheaths. The disadvantage is that they may not be as gentle or as long as you would want or need. The most common catheterization wires used for access at Children's Hospital Boston are straight wires and torque wires (both described in detail in subsequent sections) with torque wires being the more common. These have very floppy, flexible tips that allow them to find their way into small vessels quite nicely. However, you should become familiar with these expensive wires before attempting to use them since they require more technical skill and are easily damaged.

When you have your needle and wire (and catheter or sheath), you are almost ready to go, and the following sections describe access at various anatomic sites in detail. However, two common elements to access anywhere are passing your wire through your needle and exchanging your needle for your catheter or sheath.

Now, after you get that great flash of blood through your needle, you need to put a wire into the vessel. You should always use the soft end of whatever wire you have chosen (this is not always obvious with straight wires). If the wire does not go easily, it is not in the vessel. *Never, ever,* force the wire. This requires additional emphasis: *If the wire does not go easily, it is not in the vessel, and no amount of forcing it will result in success.* If a soft torque wire has one or more kinks in it when you take it out, you have pushed too hard. If the wire still does not go easily, make small readjustments to the needle position as you repeatedly try to gently advance the wire out the tip of the needle. Do *not* advance a needle over a wire because you can shear off part of the wire.

When the wire is finally in the vessel, check the position with fluoroscopy to ensure that it is where you think it should be (usually IVC to right of spine, aorta to left of spine). The color of the blood is not a sufficient marker, especially in patients on oxygen or those with cyanotic heart disease. Also, polycythemic patients may have less pulsatility on arterial hits due to the viscosity of their blood. It is better to check your position on fluoro than to put a 7 Fr sheath into the artery by accident! Just watch out for those heterotaxy patients.

Advance enough wire to have a secure position while still allowing enough of the wire outside the body to place your catheter or sheath. Do *not* advance a venous wire so far that it sends the patient into SVT (from atrial stimulation) or an arterial wire so far that it is in the brain or a coronary artery! Advance no wire so far that you lose the wire in the patient (this is considered bad form).

When the wire is in the correct position, fix the wire position relative to the patient and slide your needle off the back of the wire. You can hold the wire at the skin. There may be some bleeding around the wire before you get your sheath in. In this case you can push gently at the access site, but do not push down with such force that you bend the wire. Make a small skin nick with the blade at the wire entry site (not usually necessary for 3 Fr catheters), place the sheath/dilator combination on the back of the wire, and advance it over the wire until you see the wire coming out the back end of the sheath.

Always hold the distal wire fixed in place with the other hand. While holding near the leading end, gently twist the sheath as you advance it through the skin. Never push from the back of the sheath because this will often result in bending or kinking the sheath. Stop if there is resistance and find out why. *Never* attempt to push anything into the body when you meet resistance. After the dilator and sheath are fully advanced, remove the wire. If it is your practice, take 1 cc of blood from the (unflushed) dilator for an ACT and then remove the dilator. Flush the sheath. Avoid injecting air.

What do you do if you get a wire into the vessel but it does not advance very far? First check the wire course on fluoroscopy to make sure that it is not curled-up in the subcutaneous tissue or in a side-branch. If it appears to be in a vessel, try leaving the wire in place, removing the needle and inserting a 20-gauge IV cannula or 3 F dilator over the wire. When the cannula is in place, you can remove the wire and inject some contrast to see if the vessel is occluded. If, after you have removed the wire, you do not get blood return, you are probably not in a vessel. Do not inject contrast unless you can get blood return. When taking an angiogram, make sure to use biplane fluoroscopy. This is really the only sure way to demonstrate occlusion of the femoral or iliac vessels.

HINT: *This may seem obvious on paper, but in practice you will save yourself aggravation if you ensure that the perc needle accepts the wire you plan to use, and that the sheath or catheter you plan to use fits that wire. Until you are quite comfortable with establishing access, you should do a dry run of the needle, wire, sheath, and catheter on the table to be sure they are compatible **before** sticking the patient.*

Femoral Access

Positioning

There is not a great deal of room for error when establishing access in a tiny child. Positioning the patient is key for smooth femoral access. This is so important it bears repeating: ***Positioning the patient is key for smooth femoral access!*** Most cath lab technicians or nurses are excellent at doing this. Take note of how they do it so you can emulate their technique in the CICU and anywhere else you are called upon to place a line. The patient is appropriately then sedated and restrained. The pelvis is elevated just above the plane of the body, the femur is slightly externally rotated.

Landmarks (Figure 2)

1. *The inguinal ligament*

The inguinal ligament runs between the anterior superior iliac spine and the pubic tubercle. The inguinal ligament is your friend. Its major function is to keep the femoral arterial blood from entering the retroperitoneal space when you make a hole in the femoral artery. However, the inguinal ligament can only do its job if the hole you make in the femoral artery is *below* the ligament! Note as well that where you enter the skin is inferior to where you enter the vessels. The vessel *entry site* must be below the inguinal ligament!

2. *The femoral crease*

The femoral crease usually lies a few centimeters below the inguinal ligament. The femoral

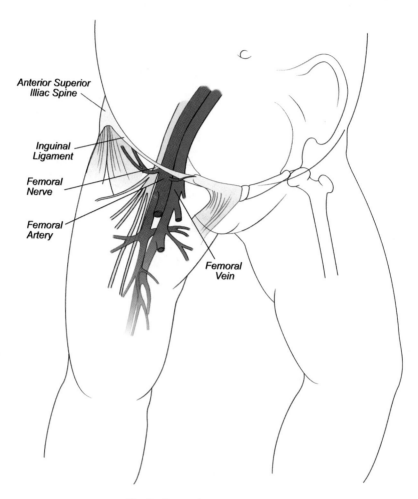

Fig. 2 Femoral access landmarks

crease is a good spot to enter the skin with the perc needle because it often lies at just the right distance from the inguinal ligament (~1 finger breadth in older children). This may not be true in adults, particularly those with weight problems.

3. *The femoral arterial pulse*

The pulse is made by the femoral artery. Always feel both sides. A pulse may feel reasonable where you are about to attempt access, but it may be bounding on the other side, suggesting that the side you are about to try on is narrowed or occluded with collateralization.

Technique

Always prep and drape both groins no matter what; it is good Karma. Feel for the femoral pulse. A *small* amount of lidocaine is infiltrated into the skin (intradermally, raising an "orange peel") and then a small amount down to the vessel to be accessed. Always withdraw on the hub of the syringe and ensure that there is not blood return prior to injecting so as not to inject lidocaine directly into a vessel. The lidocaine is massaged gently into the site to disseminate the anesthesia. Most of the pain sensation comes from the skin. Be aware that a lot of lidocaine infiltrated deep around the perc site will just make it harder to hit the vessel by distorting the anatomy or flattening the vein within the restrictive femoral sheath.

Femoral Venous Access

Usually, the venous line is placed first. An exception to this rule occurs when you have a patient in whom arterial monitoring is desired sooner rather than later.

In an older child/adult, it is usually fine to start percing just below the femoral crease at about a 30- to 45-degree angle to the skin Fig. 3. In an infant, consider percing right at the femoral crease. The femoral vein lies just medial to but touching the femoral artery. A needle angle that aims for the umbilicus is usually the right angle. Push the needle in short 1–2 mm jabs with a pause in between until you enter the vessel and blood starts flowing back in the needle hub. Short jabs are used because if you slowly and continually advance the needle you may deform the vessel, opposing the two sides, and end up perc'ing through both sides simultaneously. If you meet resistance, pull back the needle slowly *all the way to the skin*: You may have gone right through the vessel and can still get into the vessel on the way back. If suddenly you feel very little resistance, you have probably entered the pelvis! If you get

urine, someone else should probably be getting access. Do not advance the needle beyond the superior ramus of the pubis!

If the central venous pressure exceeds the atmospheric pressure plus the resistance of the needle lumen, then blood will flow from the needle hub. However, if the central venous pressure is low, you may not get any blood return even if the needle lumen is in the correct location. This is common in adults, but rare in infants. In this instance, it may be helpful to attach a syringe to the back of the needle and withdraw *gently* as you advance and then withdraw the needle. When the blood flows easily into the syringe, you are probably in the vessel. Remove the syringe, advance the wire into the vessel, and you are off to the races. To take full advantage of this technique, it is important to cut the Luer-lock off the end of the syringe or use a slip tip syringe so that it comes off easily when you need to remove it.

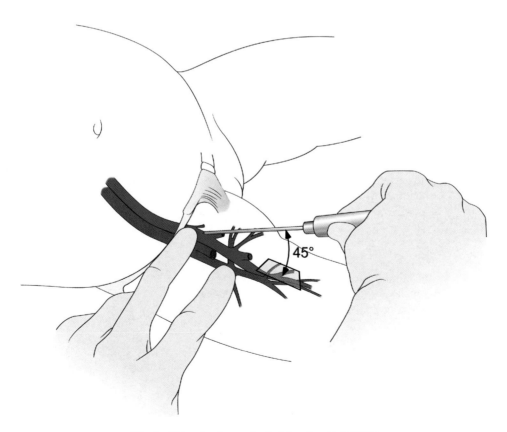

Fig. 3 Obtaining femoral arterial and venous access

Femoral Arterial Access

Accessing the femoral artery is done with a similar technique as used to access the femoral vein. Of course, the femoral artery is usually located lateral to the femoral vein just, underneath the femoral arterial pulse. The same caveats apply as before in regards to landmarks. Even more importantly, you will know when you are in the femoral artery as the blood will pulsate easily out of the vessel. If it does not, it is unlikely that you will be able to advance a wire into the femoral artery. Try to hit the femoral artery on the way in. To do this, make sure the perc needle is advanced in small short "jabs" rather than with a slow continuous motion and *not* beyond the superior ramus of the pubis. When pulsating blood returns, the hub of the needle should be brought almost parallel with the skin before the wire can be advanced. If this small motion is not made, then the wire tends to hang-up on the posterior vessel wall and may not advance up the lumen. Do not lose your cool as the blood is flying.

If you hit the femoral artery and do not succeed in cannulating the vessel, then it will often bleed and cause a hematoma. Make sure to compress the vessel until there is hemostasis before trying again.

Subclavian Vein Access

Either the left or right subclavian vein can be used; however, in practice, the left subclavian vein is usually chosen at Children's Hospital Boston because the curve to the heart and pulmonary artery is usually more favorable.

Positioning

If positioning is important for femoral access, it is even more so for subclavian access! Position the patient with the ipsilateral arm down by the side of the patient. A small towel roll between the scapulae will allow the shoulder to fall back to get it out of the way in a well-sedated patient. Be sure the shoulder is not "shrugged" as this lifts the vessel, changes the expected anatomy, and makes things much more difficult. Turn the chin away. There is no substitute for good landmarks. If necessary, you can check

fluoro to assist with difficult access, but using fluoroscopy to get access is a secondary skill and should not be used primarily.

Landmarks

Technique

A small amount of lidocaine is infiltrated into the skin and down to the clavicular periostium just lateral to the junction of the medial one-third and lateral two-thirds of the clavicle Fig. 4.

A syringe with or without a Luer Lock is placed on the hub of the needle for this access approach. The perc needle enters the skin aiming for the suprasternal notch. Get the needle just deep enough to be under the clavicle, then continue to advance the needle in a plane parallel with the floor so as to enter the subclavian vein over the first rib Fig. 5. Continuously aspirate as you advance the needle. When you enter the vein, remove the syringe from the hub of the needle, make sure it is not bright red or pulsatile,

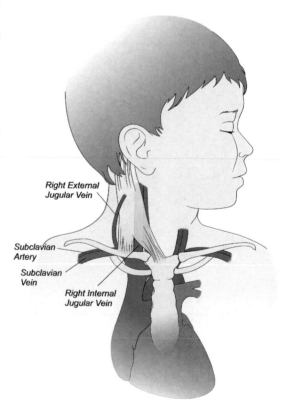

Fig. 4 Subclavian and jugular vein access landmarks

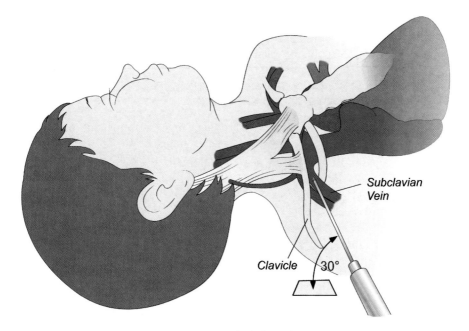

Fig. 5 Obtaining subclavian vein access

and then advance the wire. Check on fluoroscopy to ensure that the wire is taking the course that you expect. Verify that the wire is not in the subclavian artery. Place the sheath over the wire and continue.

Pointers

- The subclavian artery runs deep and cephalad to the subclavian vein. If the needle is advanced too deep to the plane of the intended target (the subclavian vein) one risks hitting the artery. A bit deeper than the artery is the pleura. Hit both and you will get a hemo/pneumothorax! Not exactly the best way to start a case.
- The subclavian vein should be entered just above the first rib to allow the puncture site to be compressed against this rib at the end of the case.
- Do not enter the left subclavian vein too medially (especially if this is a patient with a Glenn). If one enters the innominate vein, it will be difficult to do the necessary angiogram to exclude a left superior vena cava and even more difficult to get a catheter into an LSVC or other decompressing venous collateral for coil occlusion. In addition, a hemothorax is

more likely when the sheath is removed if the vessel is entered too medially.

- In a small child the sheath may advance all the way to the SVC or beyond. Catheter manipulations may require you to pull back the sheath. Be careful when performing catheter exchanges and be sure to re-advance the sheath prior to removing the catheter; otherwise you risk losing access.
- Always use a long torque wire for subclavian access. When you are sure you are in a vessel, push the wire (under fluoroscopy) until it is clearly in a venous structure (e.g., a branch PA in a Glenn or the RA, IVC, hepatic vein, or RV in a patient with an intact SVC). Follow this rule and you should never put a sheath in the subclavian artery.
- If difficulty is encountered when you are attempting subclavian access, there are two tricks that may be useful:

1. Verify the landmarks and the course of the needle fluoroscopically.
2. If there is an IV in the arm on the same side you wish to cannulate, do a venogram. To do this, put a three-way stop-cock on the peripheral IV. On one port, put 10 cc of contrast, and on the other port, 5–10 cc of saline. Ten cc's of

contrast is appropriate for an adult. For smaller children, a smaller amount of contrast should be used. If you have enough foresight, you can ask the catheterization lab nurses to try to put the peripheral IV for the cath in the arm that you want before the case even starts. Position the "camera" over the area of interest (the subclavian vein). While watching on fluoro, ask an assistant to inject the contrast, then the flush, as quickly as possible. When the contrast first becomes visible on the fluoroscopy screen, switch to the cine record pedal and you will end-up with a beautiful subclavian vein angiogram (this can, and probably should be done with store fluoro if available). Now you can use this image as a roadmap.

Internal Jugular Vein Access

Positioning

More than any other approach, successful cannulation of the internal jugular vein depends on finding the correct anatomic landmarks before starting (you may have noticed a theme here). Place a small roll under the scapulae to allow the head to fall back and expose the neck. Turn the patient's head ~ 45° to the contralateral side. Prep the area but be sure before the area is draped that the landmarks are identified because it may be more difficult to do so after the area has been draped.

To better identify the sternocleidomastoid if the patient is awake, ask the patient to lift his or her head off the table. This will contract the sterno-cleidomastoid muscle and make it much easier to identify. The right IJV is preferred over the left because the apex of the lung is lower on the right side, the path to the atrium is more direct, and there is less chance of damaging the thoracic duct.

Because there are important structures in the neck and superior mediastinum in addition to the internal jugular vein (e.g., carotid artery, trachea, and apex of the lung) it is generally a good idea to perc using a smaller needle so that less damage is done if you hit an unwanted structure. It is almost always a good idea to have a syringe on the back of your needle. Gentle suction should eliminate issues with lumen resistance and prevent an air embolus. After you enter the

appropriate vessel, advance your wire, confirm position, remove the needle, and place a sheath.

Anterior Approach

The anterior approach is useful in the intubated patient or in those whom you are expecting to place a large sheath. The entry site of the needle is lateral to the carotid artery in the middle of the triangle formed by the carotid artery, the sterno-cleidomastoid, and the mandible. Angle the needle at ~45° to the skin and aim towards the ipsilateral nipple Fig. 6.

Posterior Approach

This may seem like a strange way to enter the internal jugular vein, but it is amazingly effective in the awake patient. Identify the sternocleido-mastoid muscle by asking the patient to raise his or her head. Enter the skin inferior to the sterno-cleidomastoid muscle at the junction between the lower one-third and the upper two-thirds of the muscle Fig. 7. Avoid hitting the external jugular vein. Stay just under the muscle and aim towards the suprasternal notch (or just a bit more lateral than that). If you stay just under the muscle, then you should not hit the carotid. Note that the sternocleidomastoid muscle comes quite posterior in the older child/adult. The head may need to be turned all the way to the contralateral side in order to get behind the muscle.

Central Route

Usually this approach is avoided in the cath lab as the entry site of the vein is under the clavicle and it may be difficult to get good hemostasis after the sheath is removed. However, sometimes this approach is necessary and may preferable when placing large sheaths in small children.

Fluoroscopically Guided Approach

This technique is preferred when you already have access in one of the femoral veins and want additional venous access from the IJV. An end-hole catheter is passed from the femoral vein to the junction of the SVC and right IJV. The balloon is

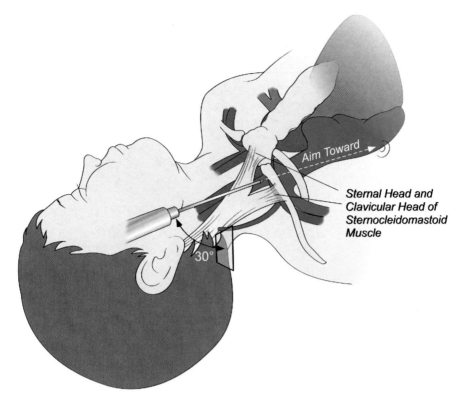

Fig. 6 Internal jugular vein, anterior approach

inflated and a small amount of contrast is placed in the vessel to define the vessel position. The perc needle enters the skin in the neck in the same position as would be used for an anterior approach and advanced towards the IJV as seen on fluoro. It may be helpful to have an assistant keep the balloon inflated on the end-hole catheter (to distend the IJ and give a bigger target) until the vessel is entered, and then deflate the balloon so it won't be punctured by the needle. NOTE: Index finger compression in the "groin" also does this for the femoral vein and artery. The wire is placed in the vessel and the sheath is placed as usual.

Ultrasound Guided Approach

In principle you can use ultrasound (US) to locate and guide access to just about any vessel, but we most commonly use ultrasound for internal jugular vein access. The process is relatively simple and is a good idea if you are unfamiliar with IJV access. There are sterile sleeves that can be used with most US probes. Once the patient is prepped and draped you can grab the probe (in the sleeve) and get a feel for the anatomy. We usually start with a quick cross-sectional look, profiling the relation of the carotid artery and internal jugular vein at the level you expect to perc Fig. 8A. The carotid usually can be seen to pulsate. If this is not immediately obvious, make sure your patient has a pulse, then try application of gentle compression by the probe. This should compress the vein but not the artery. NOTE: This is not advised in adults with atherosclerotic disease. Now center the probe on the IJV and rotate the probe 90°. This should give you a view of the IJ in the "long axis" Fig. 8B. Now you can either mentally or literally mark your trajectory and remove the probe or perc under direct US visualization.

Umbilical Vessel Access

We will not review here the technique of umbilical vessel cannulation in neonates. Using these

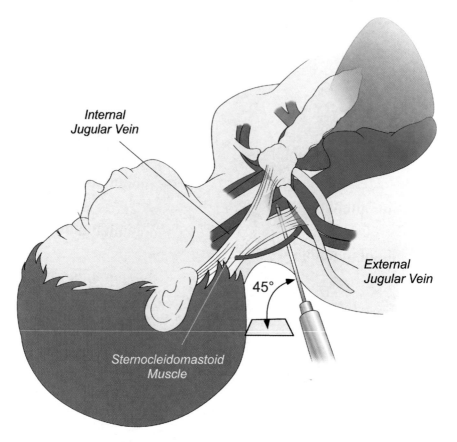

**Internal
Jugular Vein**

**External
Jugular Vein**

45°

*Sternocleidomastoid
Muscle*

Fig. 7 Internal jugular vein, posterior approach

sites for catheter access, however, deserves some attention. The usual catheters that are placed in the umbilical vessels are the 3.5 Fr or 5 Fr Argyle® umbilical vessel catheters. The 5 Fr Argyle® catheter accepts a 0.025″ in guide wire, whereas the 3.5 Fr catheter accepts a 0.021″ guide wire. If the catheters are already in-place, the area including the catheters is prepped and draped. The catheter is cut close to the skin, and the wire is advanced into the body through the catheter. The umbilical catheter is removed over the wire, and then the appropriate-sized sheath or pigtail catheter can be advanced over the wire into the body.

Ideally a regular straight wire should be used, as the shaft of a torque wire is much too stiff to be putting around the anatomic bend of the umbilical artery where it enters the internal or common iliac artery.

For umbilical venous access, it is often possible to cannulate the umbilical vein, only to encounter difficulty getting through the ductus venosus into the IVC. If this is occurring, then the catheter ends up in the portal venous system. To negotiate the ductus venosus, it is helpful to pull the umbilical catheter back into the umbilical vein and then inject a small amount of contrast, recording the injection on AP and lateral cine. The ductus venosus can then be seen and the roadmap used to negotiate a wire and catheter. You can set up a 4 F Berenstein™ with a 0.018″ or 0.014″ wire through the catheter with a sidearm of contrast filling the catheter. Insert the wire and catheter into the vein and simply inject contrast as you navigate the anatomy to the RA.

Transhepatic Access

Transhepatic access is used when there is no other venous access to the right heart, or when

(A)

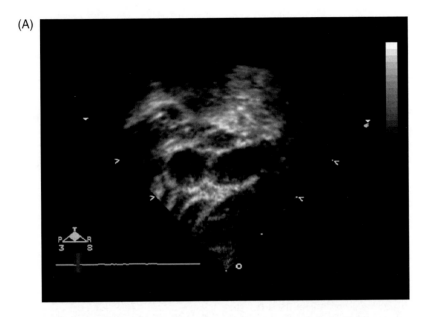

(B)

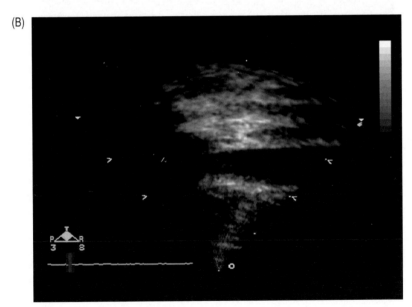

Fig. 8A, B Cross-sectional ultrasound of the right neck in a supine patient shows a round common carotid artery medially and an adjacent, slightly flattened internal jugular vein, A. After centering the probe on the IJ rotation of the probe provides a "long axis" view, B

access from below is desired for a procedure where there is no other access from below (e.g., Brockenbrough needle puncture or atrial septal defect closure in the setting of IVC occlusion).

The major risks of the procedure are damage to the liver including the bile ducts, and bleeding in the abdominal cavity. Generally, if this procedure is to be done, the patient is placed under general anesthesia to minimize patient movement. Coagulation parameters such as PT/PTT/INR should be checked during the pre-catheterization work-up.

Technique

There are two techniques for hepatic access: ultrasound-guided and fluoroscopic-guided. At Children's Hospital Boston, most cath attendings prefer to do their own transhepatic access using fluoroscopic guidance, with or without ultrasound guidance. This technique will be described below:

To make the procedure easier, if one has alternate venous access to the RA (e.g., from the right IJV), consider placing a catheter in an anterior and rightward hepatic vein and taking an angiogram to outline a good target vessel. Otherwise the procedure can be done "blindly" using anatomic landmarks.

The skin in the right subcostal region is prepped and draped. If a standard needle is too short, a 22 g Chiba® needle can be used for this access; this is a very long (15 or 22 cm), thin-walled needle with an obturator. The skin is entered just medial to the mid-clavicular line and angled quite deep to aim for the IVC-RA junction as seen on fluoroscopy. The needle is advanced on fluoroscopy. When the needle approaches the IVC-RA junction, the obturator is withdrawn and a syringe with contrast is placed on the end of the needle. The syringe is aspirated and the needle is withdrawn slowly until there is blood return. A small amount of contrast is injected to verify that the needle is in a venous vessel that returns to the heart. The syringe is removed and a 0.018″ torque-wire is passed through the needle into the vessel and (hopefully) into the RA. If the wire passes into the liver and cannot be advanced into the RA it is likely in a portal vein. In this instance the wire and needle are withdrawn and another attempt is made. After the torque wire is in the heart the needle is removed and a 5 Fr long sheath (45 cm) can be passed over the torque wire into the right atrium. If one desires a larger sheath, the wire and dilator can be removed, and a larger stiff wire passed through the sheath (e.g., a 0.035″ J-tipped Rosen®). The 5 Fr sheath can then be exchanged over the wire for a larger sheath.

The catheterization is completed as usual including routine heparinization. When finished, the tract through the liver should be closed in order to prevent bleeding. A 4 or 5 Fr Berenstein® catheter or suitable facsimile is advanced through the long sheath. The long sheath is then withdrawn to the border of the liver as seen on fluoroscopy. A small amount of contrast flushed through the side-port of the sheath will verify the position of the sheath with respect to the liver edge. The Berenstein® catheter is withdrawn while injecting contrast until the catheter is no longer in the hepatic vein but in the tract through the liver parenchyma. One or (usually) more coils about 120% the diameter of the sheath are placed into the tract to seal it (see section on coiling collaterals). When the tract is sealed, the catheter and sheath are removed.

Post-cath care consists of carefully monitoring the patient for abdominal bleeding complications. An abdominal X-ray is obtained to verify the coil position post-cath. Prophylactic antibiotics may be administered.

Angiography

Introduction

When you have your hemodynamics, you will usually proceed with angiography. Interpreting angiography correctly takes practice—lots of practice—and often this is one of the most intimidating parts of the cath experience for new fellows. You will learn it before the case (in pre-cath conference), during the case, and after (at midnight while you do your reports). You *will* learn. The following are some tips:

1. Ask. In the case, after the case, anytime.
2. When you are not cathing, try to watch cases as they happen. This is the next best thing to being in there.
3. If you see senior cardiologists reading angiograms, sit down with them. There is a bit of a time investment involved in this type of learning, but it is well worth it in many ways.

Table 1.

Frontal "Camera"		Lateral "Camera"	
Frontal/posteroanterior (PA)	0°	Straight lateral	90°
Right anterior oblique (RAO)	Usually –20–30°	Left anterior oblique (LAO)	20–70°
"Sitting Up"	0° frontal +20–30° cranial	Long axial oblique (*not* LAO)	70° lateral +30° cranial
"Laid Back"	0° frontal +30° caudal	Hepatoclavicular (4-chamber)	45° lateral +45° cranial
		Aortic orifice view	100–120° lateral +20–30° caudal

Standard Angiographic Projections

Before you can learn the standard angiographic projections you need to confront some minor confusion about the reference points for the "camera" angles. First, the "camera," such as it is, is actually an X-ray source and is *not* what people are usually referring to when they talk about imaging angles, which are commonly expressed with reference to the image intensifier or flat-panel detector (on the other side of the patient). So, while 0° is customarily called straight "AP," it is technically PA since the image intensifier is above the patient (0°) and the X-ray tube is underneath the patient (180°).

The rest is less confusing. Rotation of the image intensifier to the patient's left is considered a positive degree of rotation (also referred to as "$x°$ of

LAO"), while rotation to the right is negative (also referred as "$x°$ of RAO") Fig. 9. Cranial and caudal tilt is self-explanatory (it refers to the position of the image intensifier). Viewed from this perspective, it becomes clear why "shallow LAO" is usually between +1° and +30°, while "steep LAO" is between +61° and +89° LAO.

These angles are not set in stone. As you understand angiography better, you will make alterations from these numbers based on the patient's anatomy and on the image you are getting from the screen. Table 1 contains some basic guidelines.

When to Use Which View

Frontal/ PA View

Best used for:

- Systemic venous anatomy (RSVC, LSVC, IVC).
- Pulmonary venous anatomy.
- RV anatomy and distal PA anatomy.
- Descending aortography, aortopulmonary collaterals.
- Single ventricular morphology (especially initial imaging).

Detriments:

This is not an "axial" view. There is commonly superimposition of structures of interest. That is, the RV outflow tract overlies the branch PAs, and the ventricular and atrial septa are poorly outlined.

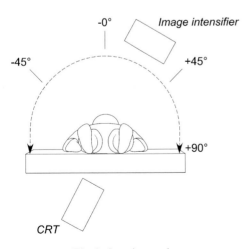

Fig. 9 Imaging angles

Right Anterior Oblique (RAO) (Fig. 10)

Superimposes normally positioned atrioventricular valve annuli. Used in electrophysiology lab for mapping.

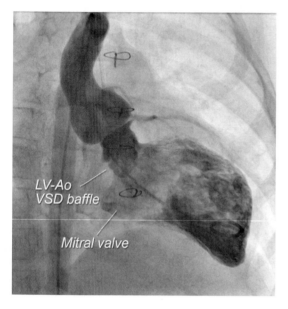

Fig. 10 RAO ventriculogram

Best used for:

- Good delineation of outlet/anterior muscular VSD's and the infundibulum.
- LV outflow tract imaging for sub-AS (including AV canal gooseneck).
- LV function and quantification of MR and AR.
- An alternative view for measuring PDAs.
- Aortic valve annulus measurements.

"Sitting Up" (Fig. 11)

Based on the old practice of moving the patient's position rather than cameras

Best used for:

- Improved imaging of MPA and branch PAs, with less superimposition.
- Pulmonary stenosis, for annulus measurements.
- Seeing full length of RPA (especially with RAO 20–30°).

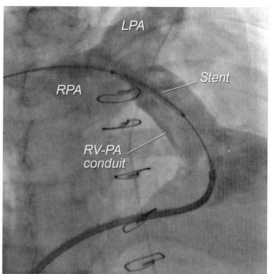

Fig. 11 Sitting up angiogram

"Laid Back" (Fig. 12)

Best used for:

- Alternate view to image proximal branch PAs.
- PAs arising from conduits (up to 60° caudal).
- Coronary arteries from Ao, e.g., D-TGA.

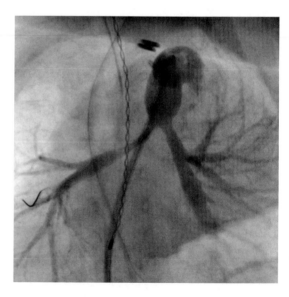

Fig. 12 Laid back angiogram

Lateral (Fig. 13)

Best used for:

- Excellent view of RV outflow tract/pulmonary valve/MPA.
- Good imaging of PDA and coarctation.
- Coronary artery origin and course.
- Distal PA anatomy.

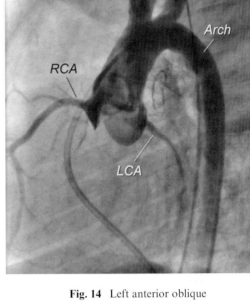

Fig. 14   Left anterior oblique

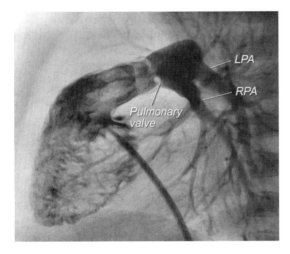

Fig. 13   Lateral angiogram

Long Axial Oblique (Fig. 15)

Gives LV image similar to that found in parasternal long axis view by echo.

Left Anterior Oblique (Fig. 14)

This is not to be confused with long axial oblique. Generally refers to the rotation along the lateral plane, and does not denote use of cranial or caudal angulation.

Best used for:

- Elongating aortic arch, which may help for PDA or coarctation,
- Lengthening LPA (caudal angulation may help),
- Truncal valve anatomy,
- Proximal LPA anatomy.

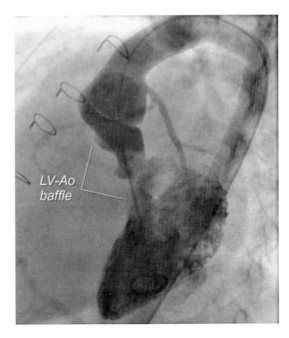

Fig. 15   Long axial oblique angiogram

Best used for:

- LV function and MR.
- Sub AS, AS, and supra-AS.
- Annulus measurement for aortic valve dilation.
- VSD imaging (membranous/conoventricular/anterior and mid-muscular).

Hepatoclavicular (4-Chamber) (Fig. 16)

Gives image analogous to that found on apical 4-chamber echo view. Looks at the crux of the heart.

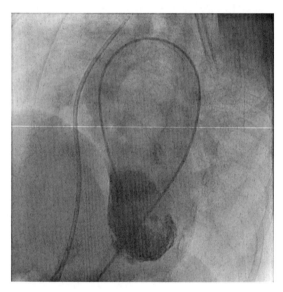

Fig. 16 Hepatoclavicular angiogram view

Best used for:

- ASDs (especially with catheter in RUPV).
- Endocardial Cushion Defects (ECD).
- Inlet/posterior muscular VSDs.
- AV valve anatomy and regurgitation.
- LV to RA shunt.
- The origin of the LPA.

Aortic Orifice View (Fig. 17)

Similar to parasternal short axis echo view.
  Best used for:

- Looking at coronary artery origins, especially with antegrade ascending aorta injection with an inflated Berman catheter.
- Gives nice view of aortic valve cusps.

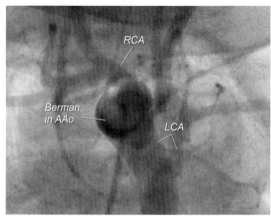

Fig. 17 Aortic orifice view

Common Catheters for Angiography

The catheters used for angiography will vary from institution to institution, and the maximum flow rates will vary by manufacturer. Listed below are several of the more common catheters, their characteristics, and the most current flow rates.

Berman[®] Catheter

This flow-directed catheter has a distal balloon, several proximal exit sideholes, and no endhole. Its use is sometimes limited by the difficulty in maneuvering it, mostly because it cannot be placed in location over a wire. There are many tricks to helping steer a Berman into position. We often shape the stiff end of a straight wire in an angle such that we can "peel off" the Berman into a desired location. Although this catheter has multiple ports for ejection of contrast, it is still important to ensure that it is not entrapped in myocardium, as it can rarely cause injury or staining in this situation, Table 2.

Table 2. Berman Catheter Sizes and Injection Rates

Size (F)	Length (cm)	Max Injection (cc/sec)
4	50	5
5	50	15
5	80	12
7	90	22

You can inflict significant harm by accidentally using an end-hole catheter for a power injection. Although we do use end-hole catheters for *hand injections* in the pulmonary arteries, coronary arteries, arterial collaterals, and venous vessels, we do not use them for any form of power-injection angiography.

Caution:

Berman catheters are very similar in appearance to pulmonary wedge end-hole catheters. You should always verify that you have the right catheter before using it or handing it to anyone. (This is critical to your survival!) This is most easily done when flushing the catheter. If flush exits via an end-hole, it's *not* a Berman.

Pigtail Catheters

This catheter is narrow-walled, made of ultrathin white teflon (i.e., the lumen is relatively large), and has numerous side-holes just proximal to the curled end. It also has an end-hole, which aids in placement over a wire. This is important, because the catheter is difficult to place in position on its own. In fact, pigtails should not be advanced without a wire, as they easily kink at the proximal side-hole. This may make the catheter prone to burst at the external junction of the hub and shaft with power injection, Table 3 outlines common sizes and injection rates. You need

Table 3. Pigtail Catheter Size and Injection Rate

Manufacturer	Size (F)	Length (cm)	Wire	Max Injection (cc/sec)
merit	3	40	0.021″	5 cc/sec
merit	3	50	0.021″	4 cc/sec
merit	4*	80	0.025″	10 cc/sec
merit	4	50	0.025″	13 cc/sec
cook	4*	70	0.035″	20 cc/sec
merit	5	100	0.035″	18 cc/sec
merit	5*	80	0.035″	20 cc/sec
cook	5*	100	0.035″	27 cc/sec
merit	6	80	0.035″	35 cc/sec
merit	6	100	0.035″	31 cc/sec
merit	7	100	0.035″	42 cc/sec

* Delivers contrast at higher flow rates for the relative size.

Table 4. Halo Catheters

Size (Fr)	Length (cm)	Max Injection (cc/sec)
4	65	20
5	65	33

to know the maximun injection rates for the catheters stocked in your lab.

We commonly use these catheters for aortograms and LV injections. They can also be guided in over a previously placed wire, which is useful when maintaining wire position is essential (such as in recently dilated pulmonary arteries or coarctations, or when you are in a difficult-to-reach position). An angiogram can be taken without removing the wire, if the pigtail is of sufficient size. Make sure the wire is securely held at the side-arm diaphragm. If this is loose, smaller wires may be injected into the patient and catheter recoil may occur with larger wires.

A cousin, the Halo catheter, can be used in similar situations, and has the added benefit of directing flow centrally, diminishing the amount of ectopy caused by the injection, Table 4.

Contrast

Type of Contrast

Historically, imaging was performed with ionic contrast, with an iodine-containing benzene ring coupled with either sodium or meglumine cations. The rates of contrast-related side effects were high, especially when using compounds with sodium salts. However, the sodium salts were less viscous, improving contrast delivery and resulting in more rapid removal from balloons. Iodine allergy is extremely uncommon as a cause for contrast reactions, because very little iodine is free in solution. Most of the problems result from rapid fluid shifts and the effects of the solutions on vascular tone.

We currently use contrast that is non-ionic, iso-osmolar and relatively low in viscosity. The non-ionic compounds have a lower rate of side effects, such as increased PA pressure, feeling of intense pain or heat on injection, and reflex tachycardia. These effects continue to be present, but to a lesser degree, and other side effects may include myocardial dysfunction, hypotension, renal dysfunction, and hyperthermia. Most of these effects are compounded by the presence of pre-existing LV dysfunction, renal impairment or small patient size.

Amount of Contrast

In patients requiring long procedures or in small babies, pre-cath planning is vital. You should be sure to take the most vital angiograms first. In some situations, you may wish to divide procedures over a couple of days. Many angiographic injection volumes will be limited by the rate of delivery for the catheter in question. This can be optimized by using the shortest catheter with the largest French size, within limits of practicality. There are no solid rules about the amount or rate of contrast delivery. People frequently quote a dose of 1 cc/kg as a guideline for most areas of the heart. However, there are several important variables that factor into the equation:

General: Higher flow rates allow for smaller contrast volumes because dye replaces un-opacified blood acutely, whereas increasing volumes at very slow flow rates are ineffective, especially in volume-overloaded lesions such as a VSD.

Patient size: It is easy to reach high levels of contrast in small patients. It may be wise to use a lower volume delivered at a faster rate to opacify the chamber in question.

Catheter location: Catheters in low flow regions (i.e., veins) do not need much contrast to get good opacification. Also, you need less contrast the further you get out into a branching vessel, such as a pulmonary artery. High volumes or rates of delivery in ventricular chambers may cause ectopy and transient AVVR.

States of high flow: You will need to increase the amount of contrast in situations of high flow or dilatation, such a ventriculograms in patients with VSDs or in other volume-loaded areas. Also, tachycardic patients may clear contrast more quickly, and generally need a larger amount of contrast. In contrast, in patients with slow heart rates, slow injection times are often sufficient and may cause less ectopy.

Layering: In some circumstances, you can decrease the amount of contrast used in hand injections by using layered injections. Because contrast is denser than NS, you can maintain separation of the two solutions in a syringe if you first draw up the saline, then the contrast (slowly), and maintain the syringe with the plunger pointed at the ceiling. This can be very useful for injections in low-flow regions, or when balloon occluding the vessel proximally.

Levophase: Levophase is the term for the phase of an angiogram (usually performed in the RV or PA) when the contrast returns from the pulmonary veins and opacifies the left heart. Levophase is your friend. You can glean a lot of information through appropriate imaging during levophase. No need to waste all of that good contrast! You should decide before starting the angiogram how long you want to image because some fluoroscopic systems time-out after a specified period of time. You should also factor increased radiation exposure into using levophase imaging.

It is better to take one good-quality image with slightly more contrast, and be able to have confidence in your diagnostic capabilities. You do not want to repeat angiograms unnecessarily or miss important information.

Minimizing Radiation Exposure (for the patient and staff members)

You will all be given a radiation safety lecture, as mandated by government regulations. Some states also require fluoroscopy licenses. Please pay attention during your training, because the pointers can be very helpful for your time in the catheterization lab. You are responsible for protecting yourself and those around you, to the best of your ability, while stepping on the fluoroscopy or cine pedal.

To remind you, here are 12 steps to reducing radiation exposure:

1. *Reduce use time*: Avoid redundant images, step off of the pedal when not acquiring a useful image, and try to use single-plane fluoro when possible. Continually ask

yourself whether you are actually using the fluoro information that you are acquiring.

2. *"Store fluoro"*: Some labs have the ability to store routine fluoroscopy as a playable loop, just like cine. If you do not need fine detail, simply step on the biplane, inject your contrast or do your intervention, step off and press "store fluoro" on the control screen.

3. *Reduce frame rate*: Available frame rates for both fluoro and cine in many labs are 7.5, 15, and 30/sec. A rate of 7.5/sec can be maddeningly stutter-like, but you can get used to it. A rate of 15/sec will provide sufficient temporal resolution for most tasks. A rate of 30/sec provides the best images, but at an obvious cost.

4. *Increase distance*: Be aware of situations where you can increase distance, such as stepping back when performing cine-angiography. Use the mobile shield, and place it between the patient and your body (not beside the lateral X-ray tube!) Make sure that other staff members are aware when a cine is about to be taken, so they can step back. Remember the inverse square law, where radiation dose is inversely proportional to the square of the distance from the source (i.e., four times less exposure at two feet vs. one foot from the source).

5. *Room lighting*: Lower ambient light levels will improve your ability to see image details, so you do not need to alter the image to do so.

6. *X-ray tube position*: Try to avoid getting direct exposure to X-rays, when possible (i.e., hands in the field). It is actually safest to stand on the left side of the patient, because most of the radiation reflects to the same side as the X-ray tube.

7. *Reduce air gaps*: A lower patient dose translates to lower operator exposure, because most occupational exposure is reflected off of the patient. You can decrease the patient dose by raising the bed as high as comfortable above the X-ray tube (the part below the table) and by lowering the image intensifier as much as possible. As an added bonus, this will also improve your image quality.

8. *Minimize magnification*: Contrary to folklore, magnification actually increases the patient dose and focuses the beam on one area, making tissue injury more likely to occur. Use only when necessary.

9. *Collimate primary beam*: Collimation is the process of bringing in dense radiation shields on the radiation source ("framing the image") and limits extraneous radiation to areas not being imaged, thereby decreasing the area of exposure for the patient. By excluding areas of vastly different density (e.g., air), the machine will not overdose the patient to improve resolution. This will also improve your image quality. You can often do this off of fluoro.

10. *Use alternate projections*: Most angled views require that the X-ray beam travel through a greater amount of tissue than the standard views, causing the machine to automatically generate more X-rays. If possible, use non-angled views.

11. *Optimize tube voltage*: Use the highest kilovolt possible to maintain adequate images. At higher kilovolt settings, more of the radiation beams pass through the patient to the image intensifier, resulting in less radiation exposure for the patient and staff.

12. *Shielding*: Wear your lead and ensure that others have theirs on before stepping on a pedal. Use the scatter shield as possible.

Catheters and Wires

There are tools for every task, and there are many tasks to be performed in the catheterization lab. The important point in pediatric and congenital cardiac catheterization is that you remain flexible with respect to the use of your tools. For example, you are more likely to use a coronary catheter to get to a PA than to actually perform coronary angiography.

You should not attempt to memorize the endless list of catheters, balloons, and devices. You should, however, be familiar with the most commonly used catheters, the general principles of these materials, and their preparation for use. The following is an introduction to catheters commonly used in pediatric catheterization

laboratories. There will be institutional variation. Expect a substantial amount of on-the-job
training).

Catheters

There are dozens of catheters in the lab, few of
which have intuitive names. It is easiest to think
of them in two large categories: end-hole catheters and angiographic catheters. End-hole catheters are used to obtain blood samples, measure
pressures in discrete locations, and selectively
cannulate small vessels such as coronaries.
When used in conjunction with a probing wire
or hand injection of contrast, they can get to
almost any location. Because they have an end-
hole, they can be exchanged over wires. Angiographic catheters have multiple side-holes over a
length of catheter. Multiple side holes allow for
delivery of a large volume of contrast rapidly,
without the creation of an end-hole jet. Although
they are great for measuring pressures as well,
they will measure the pressure over the length
of the catheter in which side-holes are present,
not at a discrete point.

Pulmonary Wedge Catheter

4 Fr-60 cm, 5-60, 5-110, 6-110, 7-110
   This is a flow-directed end-hole catheter. The
flexible shaft allows blood flow to carry the
inflated balloon naturally through the ventricle
and into the pulmonary artery. This is the catheter most commonly used at our institution for
right-sided hemodynamics, including the pulmonary capillary wedge pressure. With the balloon inflated, this catheter can also be used for
balloon occlusion pictures such as pulmonary
venous wedge pictures, innominate vein to rule
out LSVC, and so on.

Berman® Catheter

4 Fr-50 cm, 5-50, 5-80, 6-90, 7-90
   This angiographic catheter is also flow directed. It looks very similar to the wedge catheter,
but it does not have an end-hole. Proximal to the
balloon there are several holes through which
you can sample blood or inject contrast. Because

there is no end-hole, the Berman cannot be
guided to position over a wire, nor can it be
exchanged over a wire for another catheter. It
is used primarily for angiography in the ventricles where the balloon keeps the catheter away
from the myocardium, reducing the incidence of
arrhythmia, myocardial staining, and perforation during power injections. (NOTE: See angiography section for injection rates.)

Thermodilution Catheter

5 Fr, 6 Fr, 7 Fr catheters
   This is an end-hole catheter with an additional lumen terminating in a proximal side
port. There is a thermistor (temperature monitor) at the tip of the catheter, which aids in
cardiac index assessment using cold saline injections via the proximal port. On the 5 Fr catheters
the proximal port is 15 cm from the tip (generally
used in children <15 kg), and in the 6 Fr and 7 Fr
catheters, the proximal port is 29 cm from the
tip. The two small lumens not only make it a
poor catheter for transducing pressures, they
also make the catheter relatively stiff. The end-
hole lumen accepts only a very small guide wire,
so for positioning you are mainly at the mercy of
this stiff, flow-directed catheter.

Double Lumen Wedge Catheter

7 Fr
   These catheters have the standard end-hole
that can be used for pressure readings and for
the taking of samples. In addition, there is a
second port for pressure recording at 1 cm in
the 5 Fr catheter, 2 cm in the 6 Fr catheter, and
3 cm in the 7 Fr. The double lumens allow for the
simultaneous measurements of two areas of
pressures, such as transchamber pressure measurements, and can be used to record pressure
gradients across valves.

Multipurpose Catheter

4 Fr, 5 Fr, 7 Fr
   The multipurpose catheter is a relatively
stiff end-hole catheter that has a terminal
bend. In addition to the end-hole, there are
two side-holes near the tip Fig. 18. This

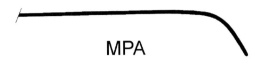

Fig. 18 Multipurpose catheter

catheter is versatile, as its name implies, and can be used for many tasks including right heart cath, probing the atrial septum, pressure measurements over a wire, angiography by hand, and so on. Generally, it is not recommended for coil placement unless the tip with the side-holes is cut off.

Berenstein® Glide Catheter

4 Fr 0.035″ 5 Fr 0.038″

The Berenstein is a soft, low-torque, end-hole catheter that has a small bend on the end. Using this catheter and probing with the floppy end of the torque wire, one can get into most branch vessels, collaterals, etc. Because they track small wires well, but accept a much larger wire, they are extremely useful for multiple catheter exchanges. They can also be used for coil delivery.

Bentson® Glide Catheter

4 Fr 0.035"

The Bentson is also a relatively soft, low-torque endhole catheter with a bent end and a large secondary curve Fig. 19. It is also used to enter small vessels or advance wire position. The primary bend can help to stabilize the catheter. The Bentson can also be used for coil delivery.

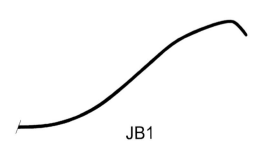

Fig. 19 Bentson catheter

Cobra Catheter

4 Fr, 5 Fr, 7 Fr

The Cobra has a larger secondary curve than the Bentson catheter, directing the tip of the catheter more than 90° back toward the primary direction of the shaft Fig. 20. This curve provides it with greater stability of position along some tortuous catheter courses; however, it does not track as well as the Bentson or the Berenstein.

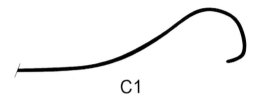

Fig. 20 Cobra catheter

Judkins Right and Left Coronary Catheters

4–7 Fr with 1–5 curves

The coronary catheters are designed to get into the corresponding coronary artery. The choice of curve depends on the width and length of the aortic arch Fig. 21 and 22. They can also be used for entering a variety of collaterals or shunts. The tips can be cut to customize the curvature and reach, but care should be taken not to create sharp catheter tips, which may cause vascular damage.

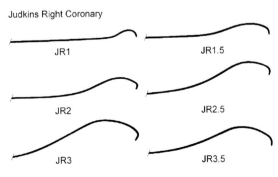

Fig. 21 Judkins right catheters

Judkins Left Coronary

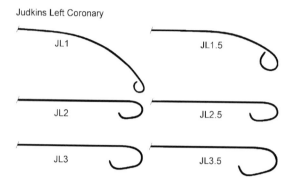

Fig. 22 Judkins left catheters

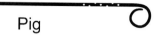

Pig

Fig. 24 Pigtail catheter

Amplatz Right and Left Coronary Catheters

4.5–7 Fr with curves AR1 and Ar2 or AL2 and Al3

The Amplatz catheters are also designed for entry into the coronary arteries Fig. 23. Again, we frequently cut these catheters for customized curves and reaches for catheter-directed access to various locations.

Pigtail Catheters

3–7 Fr with lengths of 40–110 cm

These are generally considered angiographic catheters, due to their ultra-thin walls and multiple side-holes Fig. 24. Although they do have an end-hole, the pigtail shape and the taper of the catheter down to the end-hole prevent a terminal jet of contrast when large volumes of contrast are injected rapidly. You must still take care to keep the end of the pigtail out of smaller vessels such as coronary arteries during power injections, as a forceful jet of contrast can still cause injury. They will track a wire, and should be advanced over a wire in order to prevent

kinking of the pigtail. The pigtail will automatically reform when the wire is removed. The multiple side-holes are all positioned close together to give single-chamber injection. They are used for angiography in the ventricles (especially the LV) and the ascending aorta, and they are good for pressure measurements as well. Each individual French size and length combination has its own maximal burst pressure (be aware of the injection rate for the pigtail you are using), above which the catheter does actually burst at the junction of the shaft and hub (generally all over the fellow!).

There are pigtails that have radiographic markers of distance and size, which allow them to be used to more accurately determine angiogram magnification. They can also be used for angiograms themselves, but they are made from a stiffer material so that they generally do not tolerate as large a volume and flow rate as the same-sized regular pigtail. The marker pigtails are often not used for angiography. but are placed somewhere else in the field to provide a reference for measurements.

When the tip of a pigtail catheter is cut off, the catheter becomes much less curved, and the end-hole becomes larger, so there is room for contrast to exit the end-hole even if there is a wire present. This modification is extremely important, and was made so frequently in our lab that a former fellow actually convinced the manufacturer to make a "Cut-off Pig" and got his name put on the catheter! (discontinued recently) Cut pigtail catheters will track a stiff wire relatively well. When in position, a Y-adapter

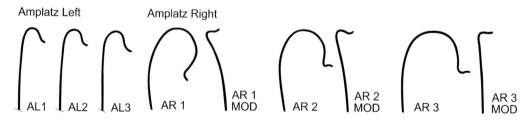

Fig. 23 Amplatz catheters

allows you to measure pressure and take pictures using the multiple side-holes and the end-hole. The presence of the wire prevents a terminal jet.

Wires

Wires serve three basic functions: probing, guiding, and exchanging. All wires have a stiff end and a soft end. Most of the time, the soft end of the wire is the business end. In some situations, the stiff end of the wire can be very useful, but it must not be advanced into the body alone. *Beware*: Advancing the stiff end of wire out the end of a catheter risks perforating the heart or vessel, or more commonly lifting an intimal flap.

The guide wire is a vital part of the catheterization procedure. A perfect guide wire would be strong enough to allow catheters to track over it without kinking. It would be steerable and have a floppy torqueable tip. In addition, it needs to be radio-opaque. All guide wires really consist of two parts: a mandrel core and a spring guide that is wrapped around it. The mandrel is a solid wire that runs the length of the wire. It can be fixed or moveable. If it is fixed, the core is welded to both ends of the outer coil Fig. 25. The moveable mandrel is only welded at one end. The mandrel can then move in relation to the end of the spring guide changing the stiffness of the tip of the wire (this is true for most J wires).

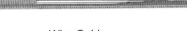

Wire Guide
TFE coated stainless steel

Fig. 25 Wire core

Straight Wires

These wires have, as the name suggests, a soft, straight tip. These are the wires that are used for arterial access, for advancing pigtail catheters, and so on. They are relatively good, cheap guide wires. Although the tips are soft, these wires are

Table 5. Sizes and Lengths of Straight Wires

Wire	House	Length (cm)
0.018″	Green	145
0.021″	Black	145
0.025″	Blue	145
0.035″	Purple	145
0.038″	Red	145

not "floppy" and they are not very good for probing for vessels. They are not very long, and so are not ideal for catheter exchanges. The stiff end of the wire will hold any bend you give it, so these wires can be shaped and used to guide catheters through relatively simple courses. These wires come in a variety of sizes and lengths, Table 5.

Torque Wires

The torque wires have a stiffer mandrel than the straight wires. The core is made of stainless steel, and the tip is made of platinum, making it very radio-opaque. The last few centimeters are extremely shapeable. The floppy end has great steerability and great torquing capabilities. The torque wires are available in 0.018″ (blue case) and 0.035″ (purple case), Table 6.

Table 6. Torque Wires

Wire	Length (cm)	House
0.018″	145	Blue
0.035″	180	Purple
0.035″ "exchange"	260	Purple

ThruWay® Wire

0.018", 190 cm

These wires are much like the usual 0.018" wire; however, this wire is a bit longer and can be used as an exchange wire for most catheters and balloons taking a 0.018" wire. There is a 5-cm tapered "floppy" end, with the remainder of the wire being moderately stiff.

V-18 Control Wire®

0.018″, 200 cm

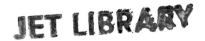

The V-18 is somewhat similar to the 0.018"
torque wire. It has an 8-cm flexible tip with a
hydrophilic coating. It is 200 cm long and the
remainder of the wire is quite stiff which makes
exchanges easier, but it also requires fairly precise preshaping to not distort cardiac or vascular
structures.

Cook Deflecting Wire

The deflecting wire has a movable core, that is,
the mandrel is only fixed at one end and the
spring guide can move along it. These wires
come out of their houses straight. At the stiff
back end, they have two steel markers, which
are used to seat the wire into the handle. These
also come preassembled Table 7 and Fig. 26.
When the wire is in a position in the heart
where you would like it to bend, you pull the
trigger on the handle and it progressively bends
the wire by pulling the steel markers apart from
each other. Often, after the catheter is pointing
in the desired direction, the catheter can be
advanced into the desired position. The distal
tip of the wire is quite stiff and should not be
advanced out of the catheter. When using the
deflector, it is very easy to break the distal end
when applying a lot of pressure especially the
0.025".

Table 7. Cook Deflecting Wire

Wire Size	Length (cm)	Radius of Curve (mm)
0.025"	125	5
0.035"	145	5

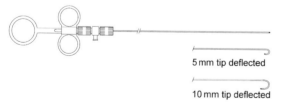

5 mm tip deflected

10 mm tip deflected

Fig. 26 Cook wire

Rosen® Wire

0.035", 220 cm

The Rosen wire is an exchange-length wire. It is
a long wire with a heavy-duty mandrel to within
2 cm of the tip, making it a very good tracking
wire. The soft tip is flexible with a "J" on the end,
Fig. 27. This wire is very useful for PA dilations.
The catheter comes with a little purple introducer
to help you get the J tip into the hub of your
catheter. You will invariably lose the introducer
or not have enough time to put it back on the wire
before you are expected to put the wire through a
catheter. A neat trick is that if you pull back on the
part right after the "J" the tip will straighten out
and you will be able to load the wire.

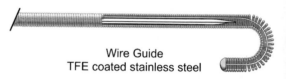

Wire Guide
TFE coated stainless steel

Fig. 27 Rosen wire

Amplatz Super Stiff® Wires

0.025" and 0.035" 260 cm

This is another exchange-length wire. It is very
long, making it possible to exchange long catheters or sheaths over them in even the tallest
patients. The Amplatz wires are great guide
wires because they are very stiff. The inner mandrel is large and the exterior coil wire is flattened,
causing the wire to be very strong. The distal ends
are relatively soft. These wires can be bent into
shape and continue to hold that shape after being
passed through a floppy catheter. They have very
good trackability, even when bent. They are often
used for angioplasty of difficult-to-reach sites
with difficult bends. Because of their stiffness,
they can cause hemodynamic problems related
to propping open traversed valves.

Stabilizer® Wire

0.014", 300 cm

Although many 0.014" wires exist, the stabili-
zer wire is the only exchange length wire carried at
Children's Hospital Boston in an 0.014" size.
They are very hard to see when on the table.

They are incredibly long as well–300 cm (because they have to make it all the way to the adult coronary arteries). Your challenge will be to find them and then load them with balloons in a dimly lit cath lab. Also, you will need to try very hard to distinguish them from the 0.014″ seeker wires.

How to Hold a Wire

You will spend a great deal of time holding wires during cases. As you might suspect, this provides many opportunities for mishap. We offer the following tips to aid you in your experience.

Try to keep track of what wires you have, and organize them on the table while the case is proceeding. When wires are removed from the body it is your job to wipe them down with gauze dipped in the flush. This will take the blood off of the wires and make them less sticky. Try to put the wires back in their houses if they are not going to be reused immediately. This will help hours later when there are 12 wires on the table. Be sure you don't put away a wire that is still in the patient!

Half of your time will be spent getting wires into tricky places. The other half will involve placing catheters in or removing them over the wire. The goal here is not to lose wire position. Losing wire position is one of the worst things you can do in the cath lab. The seriousness of this offense increases exponentially in relation to the time that it took to get to that vessel. Of course, the harder it was to get to that vessel, the easier it is to lose wire position.

So, let's start with getting a catheter removed over the wire. A wire will finally be in whatever position you need it, after you have spent some interminable time getting there. Now you need to take a catheter out over this wire so you can advance a new catheter (often a balloon).

To remove a catheter over a wire, you need to use both hands; one goes on the wire, the other on the catheter. Your eyes (it is hard to believe at first, but it is true) need to be **on the screen** watching the tip of the wire. Do not look at your hands! You will place the hand on the wire a short distance from the hand on the end of the catheter and then pull the catheter until it meets the other hand. (If you only look at your hands, you will move the tip of the wire even though it does not seem like you did.) It usually helps to rest your wire hand on the table, for a

point of stability. You then reposition the wire hand and repeat this maneuver until the person at the groin (usually the attending) says they have the wire. When they have the wire securely in their hands, one of you can then pull the catheter the rest of the way off the wire a bit more quickly. If you are alone, you can do this as well, but it will probably take a while longer.

So now the wire is going through the sheath to somewhere you are very interested in, and you need to get something (another catheter) over the wire. Many catheters are relatively stiff and sometimes give you trouble going around the turns that the wire traverses, but you are going to get your catheter there. Your first job will be to place the catheter on the tip of the wire. Usually, especially when you are new, the attending will be holding the end of the wire near the sheath through this procedure, but it is your responsibility to see if anyone is holding the wire. *Always* know if someone is holding wire. Your catheter can be loaded either way, but you need to adjust your methods a little and be a bit gentler if no one is holding the other end of the wire.

You place the catheter on the free end of the wire and then you need to advance the catheter until you see the wire come out the back end. When you have the end of a wire in your hand, ensure that the wire is being held near the sheath, and then pull the wire taut. It is very important while you are pulling the wire taut that you do not also advance the catheter: *This will cause you to lose wire position.* When you have the wire taut (often you should plant your hand on the table to be sure it does not move), the catheter can be advanced forward, Fig. 28.

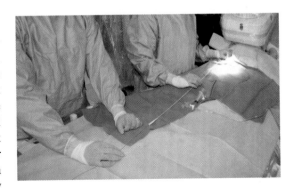

Fig. 28 Holding a wire

Generally, you want to hold the wire until the catheter is exactly where you want it, but there are times when you need to let go of the wire. How do you tell the difference? Again, you need to be looking at the screen. Occasionally, when you hit a certain curve the catheter will get hung up. If you continue to push the catheter the tip of the wire will start to come back; this is the point when the attending will "vigorously instruct" you to let go of the wire. Let go. From here you can either advance wire or push both to allow the wire to move forward. As you get used to it, you will be able to tell when this is happening and let the wire go at the right time. You can often feel this when you are the one advancing the catheter.

The other problem that can happen is that the wire can be advanced with the catheter. This generally means that you are not holding the wire tight enough, although it can happen when a stiff catheter straightens out the more curved course that the wire was taking. If you are watching the screen, you can adjust the wire to compensate for this. Otherwise you will get "firm suggestions" to hold the wire or move the wire. You will repeat this procedure many times in every case, especially when dilating pulmonary arteries.

You will have to hold wires sometimes when inflating balloons. This is usually when there is risk that the balloon will be milked forward with the dilation thereby also pushing the wire forward, particularly with valve dilations. Pushing the wire forward is not a good thing because you don't know where it will go, especially if you already have it in a small branch pulmonary artery. The wire's shape is also distorted with dilation. These two things combined can cause quite a bit of damage to the small distal vessels.

Another time you commonly will be holding the wire is when you take an angiogram through a pigtail that is over a wire. You need to hold the wire and the Y-connector firmly—the wire so that it is not also injected forward with the power injection, and the Y-connector because they break a lot.

At the End of the Case

At the end of the case, it is time to pull the lines. If you have sheaths in both the artery and vein you can just pull the sheaths without any other manipulation. If, however, you have a pigtail catheter (or other shaped catheter) in a vessel (or still in the sheath), you should remove the catheter over a wire (the soft end of a straight wire will do), taking care that the wire straightens out the catheter such that when you pull both out neither the wire nor the catheter damage the vessel by being "hooked" around the sheath or vessel wall.

Balloons, Stents, and Devices

The available catheterization lab armamentarium is ever changing, and varies not only over time but also from institution to institution. The following section describes general principles on the use of the most common of these items at the time of this writing.

Balloons

Selected Terminology and General Principles

Balloon Profile: The diameter of the deflated balloon

- Dictates sheath requirements.

Balloon Length: The length of the parallel portions of the inflated balloon (does not count the taper).

- Long balloons improve stability during inflation; often preferred in dilation of aortic valves in older children. They take longer to inflate and deflate fully.
- Short balloons cause less straightening of curved cardiac or vascular structures, and thus may cause less injury at the tips of the balloon.

Compliance: The degree of stretch at low pressure.

- Very compliant balloons preferentially enlarge within the normal part of the vessel, applying less pressure to the stenotic segment. These balloons may tear or rupture the normal vessel with minimal dilation of the stenosis.
- Noncompliant balloons increase their diameters more equally across the stenotic lesion and normal vessel.

- Noncompliant balloons have more predictable maximum inflation diameters compared to compliant balloons.
- Very compliant balloons are primarily used for sizing defects.
- Noncompliant balloons are preferred for stent placement or tight stenoses.

Dilating Radial Force Vector (tight waist vs. shallow waist):

- If the balloon diameter is small compared to the lesion, only a subtle waist is produced and the dilating force is small. The dilating force can be increased by increasing the inflation pressure, but this puts the balloon at risk for rupture.
- If the balloon diameter is large compared to the stenosis, the waist will be very tight and the dilating force will be large. In this setting, the normal vessel (proximal and distal to the stenosis) is at greater risk of injury. Also, when the balloon is under pressure, when the vessel begins to tear, it will rapidly tear all the way to the full balloon diameter (i.e., the bigger the balloon, the deeper the tear).
- Intermediate waists are the most effective and safest for nearly all lesions. Visualizing the waist and reacting appropriately is one of the most important skills in interventional cardiology.
- During inflation, the dimensions of the waist must be determined and a decision made whether or not to fully inflate the balloon. As a general rule, if the waist is < 75% the diameter of the proximal and distal balloon, it is too tight; the balloon should not be fully inflated, and the dilation should be repeated with a smaller balloon.

Sample Balloon Inventory and Specific Characteristics

See the Appendix. (p. 155–162)

Preparing a Balloon and Using a Gauge

You will prepare a thousand balloons during your fellowship. Try to modify your technique each time based on the specific needs of the case you are doing.

CAUTION: *Inappropriate balloon preparation can result in poor balloon visualization, air embolism or prolonged circulatory occlusion.*

How to Prep a Balloon

Remove the catheter from the packaging using sterile technique, and lay it on the table. To prepare the balloon, a 10-cc syringe (for balloons less than 10 mm) or a 20-cc syringe (for larger balloons) is filled with a combination of contrast and saline. The ratio of contrast to saline differs for each type of balloon and intervention. For small coronary balloons and cutting balloons less than 4 mm, the syringe should be highly concentrated with contrast, nearly 100%, so it will be easily visible by fluoroscopy. As the size of the balloon increases, and therefore the depth of contrast material in the balloon increases, adequate visualization can be achieved with more dilute mixtures. A typical mixture for, say a 5–10 mm balloon, is one-third contrast and two-thirds saline. A high concentration of contrast increases the viscosity of the fluid and therefore the inflation and deflation times of the balloon (long inflation/deflation times are unwise if you are obstructing cardiac output, e.g., dilating an aortic valve). However, the balloon will be easily seen, and any waist in the balloon will be easier to appreciate. A low concentration of contrast will flow into and out of the balloon more readily, but may make it difficult to see a waist.

A syringe with the appropriate amount of contrast/saline is attached to the balloon lumen of the catheter. The balloon lumen is always the one that comes off the shaft at an angle. It is also marked "balloon." The other lumen is the end-hole lumen, and should be flushed with saline. After the syringe is on the balloon lumen, pull the plunger back and lock it—three times if you have time. The syringe is locked by pulling the plunger to the end of the syringe until it "catches," and it will maintain some negative pressure without being pulled on. Between pulls, tap the hub of the balloons to free up any air bubbles that have been withdrawn. **Do not** push the plunger. This will start to inflate the balloon and increase its profile, making it more difficult to get into the body and to the dilating site. After you have fully prepped the balloon, leave the syringe locked and get the tip of the catheter in your hand, ready to load on the guide wire.

Using a Gauge

Gauges allow you to apply a specific amount of inflation pressure. Generally, hand inflation is ≤ 8 ATM, although obviously the stronger you are and harder you push, the higher the pressure (a hard push can approach 12–14 ATM). If you are pushing hard. it is a good idea to know how hard, and for that we use a gauge.

There are many varieties of gauges, but they all work in a similar manner. Most allow you to freely push the plunger, then lock the plunger and twist a handle that gradually increases the pressure. A manometer allows you to follow your progress. To use a gauge you first have to prep it. This essentially means filling it with saline and/or contrast. The ratio of saline to contrast depends on whether you intend to start inflation with the gauge or with a prepped balloon and then swap out for a gauge. If you are starting with a gauge, fill it with a saline/contrast ratio as you would a syringe for the balloon. If you are just swapping in the gauge after the balloon is essentially fully inflated with contrast, then the ratio in the gauge matters less because little will actually enter the balloon.

When you have locked the gauge, start turning the handle clockwise to increase the pressure. Call out your inflation pressures. You cannot usually simultaneously watch the screen and the manometer, but try and also listen carefully to your attending to tell you when to stop. When you are ready to deflate the balloon, you can just turn the plunger counterclockwise, but this takes forever. Instead, it is much quicker to unlock the gauge and pull back as you would a normal syringe. Then you can lock the gauge with negative pressure. Remember that some gauges have no backstop on the plunger, so you can easily pull the plunger all the way out and lose all of your negative pressure. *Don't do this.* If you do, the easiest solution is to disconnect the tubing from the catheter and attach a standard 10-cc syringe to the catheter, pull it back, and lock it. This empty syringe should always be easily accessible for any balloon dilation/deflation.

Optimal Balloon Selection: Lesion

NOTE: *The following are guidelines. The ultimate decision to inflate a balloon is based on the appearance of the waist as it begins to form in the lesion.*

Coarctation of the Aorta

- Initial balloon diameter 2.5–3× the diameter of the coarctation.
- At most, 120% of the diameter of the aorta proximal and distal to the coarctation.
- Shortest balloon available (2 cm for infants/children; 3–4 cm for adolescents).
- Smallest possible arterial or venous sheath size (low-profile balloon).
- Higher inflation pressures and high-pressure balloons are often needed for re- coarctations (less compliant lesions)

Branch Pulmonary Artery Stenosis/Hypoplasia

- Initial balloon diameter 3–4× the lesion diameter.
- $\leq 2\times$ the diameter of the normal distal PA.
- Adjust the balloon size to the degree of waist observed during dilation.
- Prefer short balloons with minimal tip length (short taper).
- High-pressure balloons usually preferred.

Homograft/Conduit Stenosis

- Balloon diameter up to 110% of the implanted conduit diameter.
- Prefer shorter balloons to minimize straightening of calcified conduit.
- High-pressure balloons are required.
- Stenting frequently necessary.

Pulmonary Valve Dilation

- Balloon diameter 120–130% of the annulus (lateral view, RV angiogram).
- 2 cm long for infants/young children; 3–4 cm for older children/adults.
- Low-profile balloon and short taper are an important feature for newborns.

- For critical PS in neonates: initial balloon 2–4 mm, 1 cm long; then dilate up to 120–130% of the measured valve annulus.

Aortic Valve Dilation

- Initial balloon diameter 80–90% of the valve annulus (LV angio; long axial oblique and RAO).
- Valve damage increases significantly at balloon: annulus ratio ≥ 1.10.
- Stiff guide wire and longer balloons help stabilize the balloon across the valve.
- Low-profile balloons allow smaller sheath sizes.

Mitral Valvotomy

- A general guide to initial balloon sizing is based upon BSA:
  - 8 mm in patients $\leq 0.4\,m^2$
  - 10 mm in patients ~ 0.4–$0.8\,m^2$
  - 12 mm in patients ~ 0.9–$1.2\,m^2$
  - 15 mm in patients $\geq 1.2\,m^2$
- Adjustments in balloon diameter are made according to waist on inflation.

Stents

Indications

Intravascular stents have been used in children since 1989. Specific indications include lesions unresponsive to conventional balloon dilation (compliant obstructions, stenoses due to kinking, external compression or intimal flaps), stenotic anastomoses in the early postoperative period, recanalized vessels/baffles or thrombosed shunts, and following significant tears or aneurysmal formation during balloon angioplasty.

CAUTION: *Stents are not well suited for a number of situations, either because of lack of efficacy or undesirable characteristics.* Some of these include:

- Stent placement in young children is avoided when possible. With newer, higher-pressure balloons, some stents may be broken, but at this point it remains wise to not rely upon this.

- Stents within stenoses in the distal pulmonary arteries often cover and may obstruct side branches.
- Stents placed within pulmonary veins usually produce good immediate results; however, restenosis and occlusion can be anticipated within weeks to months.
- Stents placed across the transverse aortic arch may cover and possibly obstruct brachiocephalic vessels.

Stent Inventory

Stent inventory will vary from institution to institution. We currently carry four types of bare metal stents, which roughly divided by size, are:

1. Coronary Express® stents (Boston Scientific)
2. Palmaz Genesis® pre-mounted stents (Cordis);
3. Palmaz Genesis® XD stents (Cordis) Fig. 29
4. Palmaz XL stents (Cordis) Fig. 30
5. Palmaz Blue® stents (Cordis)
6. ICAST® pre-mainted covered stents (ATRIUM)

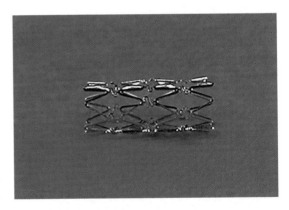

Fig. 29 Genesis stent

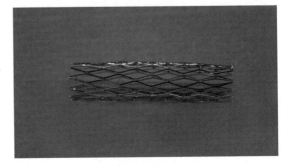

Fig. 30 Palmaz stent

Each type of stent has its own set of characteristics, with advantages and disadvantages, which are beyond the scope of this manual. You should know that some stents "shorten" in length the more they are dilated, so be aware of the stent characteristics prior to placement.

Covered Stents

There are a variety of premade balloon-expandable and self-expanding covered stents on the market. Additionally, "hand-made" stents can be prepared by sewing surgical Gortex Gore-Tex® into a cylinder of a required diameter and then attaching this to the outside of a stent of the desired size. This requires some know-how and is not advised for the inexperienced. Some indications for covered stents include simultaneous dilation of baffle obstruction and closure of baffle leak/fenestration, closure of a Potts' shunt or aortopulmonary window, vessel recanalization and as rescue for significant vascular injury.

How to Load and Deliver a Stent

After it has been determined that stent placement is appropriate, a stent size is chosen based on the balloon size used for dilation and the desired final size of the vessel. The length of the stent is decided upon based on location of the stenosis and the risk of compromise of adjacent vessels. In general, we choose the shortest possible stent that is likely to address the stenosis.

If you do not have an appropriate premounted stent available you must mount it yourself. Traditionally, a stent is hand-crimped onto a balloon that is delivered through a long sheath that has previously been positioned across the lesion. A front-loading technique can be used as well.

Equipment

Balloons

- The balloon profile should be large enough to prevent slipping of the stent.
- Scratch-resistant balloons minimize the risk of balloon rupture.
- Nonslippery/hydrophobic balloons minimize stent instability during inflation.

- Longer balloons maximize stent stability during expansion.
- Shorter balloons reduce the risk of the stent puncturing the balloon, especially if the course involves a curve.

Wires

- Depends on the balloon/stent being used. For large stents one of the following:

  o 0.035″ Rosen—moderately stiff/curved end—usually used if the wire course is relatively straightforward.
  o 0.035″ Super Stiff®–very stiff/soft end—provides more stability; must be pre-bent to conform to bends within the heart or vasculature.

Procedure and Techniques

Back Loading

A stiff wire (e.g., Amplatz Super Stiff) is secured in position across the area to be stented. Shaping the wire to accommodate the curves during its course is helpful in stabilizing its position. The long sheath and dilator are then advanced over the wire to beyond the area of stenosis. A balloon catheter is chosen for stent delivery. Be sure the balloon shaft is longer than your long sheath! Before the dilator of the sheath is removed, the balloon must be prepared. If the long sheath lacks a hemostasis valve, some sort of side arm or adapted short sheath must be placed on the balloon catheter shaft, preferably before the stent is crimped on it. The dilator is then withdrawn slowly and the balloon/stent/side arm apparatus is loaded onto the wire and into the long sheath. The balloon/stent is then advanced over the wire until the stent is centered across the area of stenosis.

If there is difficulty advancing the balloon/stent the last few millimeters around a curve in the sheath, the entire apparatus may be moved forward. The sheath is then pulled back off of the balloon, remembering to allow some distance for the balloon taper. A hand injection can be done through the side port of the long sheath to confirm stent position relative to the lesion, and then the balloon is inflated and stent delivered. If the stent has slipped back on the balloon during positioning, the balloon can be partially inflated to release the stent into the vessel, and the end of the sheath used to buttress the stent while the balloon catheter is deflated and pulled back to straddle the stent. The procedure is then continued with full inflation of the balloon deploying the stent in position. The balloon catheter is then removed and the results are assessed, with the possibility of re-dilating the stent with a larger balloon or to flare poorly apposed ends.

Front Loading

Front loading is an alternative technique. It involves placement of a stent directly in the distal aspect of the long sheath. In this technique the balloon catheter carrying the stent acts as the dilator for the long sheath as it is passes up to and through the stenosis. Because the balloon and stent do not have to travel through the long length, and possibly multiple curves, of the long sheath, this technique decreases the likelihood of stent "slippage" during delivery. It also generally allows a slightly smaller long sheath, as there is not as much need for room around the balloon/ stent within the sheath. However, unless the balloon tip is to be passed bare through the groin, it does not end up saving much in terms of sheath size in the groin.

An exchange length wire (Rosen or Amplatz Super Stiff)is placed in the desired position. The long sheath is flushed. A short sheath that will accommodate the long sheath is chosen (1–2 sizes larger) and their compatibility is tested. The short sheath is inserted into the site of venous access over the guide wire. The desired balloon is advanced through the long sheath until it extends beyond the end of the sheath. The stent is mounted on the center of the balloon by compression with moderate pressure; rolling between the fingers. Avoid severely crimping the ends of the stent, which may puncture the balloon. The proximal and distal portion of the balloon can be sequentially partially expanded while compressing the opposite end of the balloon to assure equal trouble free inflation of each end

of the balloon. This can be crucial for stent stability during inflation because if only one end expands it can "milk" the stent off the balloon.

The stent/balloon combo is then withdrawn into the end of the long sheath without dislodging the stent (this is usually a tight fit). Check to see that the stent/balloon combo comes out of the sheath smoothly by advancing the balloon catheter out enough to partially uncover the stent. Leave about 1 cm of the balloon catheter tip extending beyond the end of the sheath for smooth transit through the heart. The balloon/ stent/long sheath combo is then advanced over the guide wire through the short sheath (or skin). Take care to keep the relationship of the balloon catheter and the long sheath constant by holding both together at the hub of the sheath. Advance the combo to the area of interest. When the stent is appropriately positioned the long sheath can be pulled back leaving the stent position unchanged. Hand injections of contrast through the sidearm of the long sheath are valuable in assessing stent position and should be recorded for use as reference images. The position is adjusted as necessary.

Peri-Stent Care

Specific recommendations are included in the sections on typical lesions. In general:

- Although general anesthesia is not usually required, stent implantation requires sufficient sedation so as to eliminate patient movement.
- We usually recommend that an appropriate antibiotic be administered.
- The ACT should be maintained at > 200 during the procedure.
- Unless specifically contraindicated, a Heparin infusion should be considered overnight for stents in low-flow areas (Fontan baffles, pulmonary vessels, etc.)
- Consider anticoagulation therapy asprin, plavise, or coumadin as appropriate.
- CXR (PA/Lateral) should be reviewed post-catheterization to assess stent position and integrity

Complications

Embolization

This is one of the most feared complications as it may require surgical removal. If the stent is not secure after it is expanded, re-expanding the balloon in the stent and maneuvering the balloon/stent combination proximally may allow fixation of the stent in another portion, or in non obstructive position in the systemic venous system, Fig. 31.

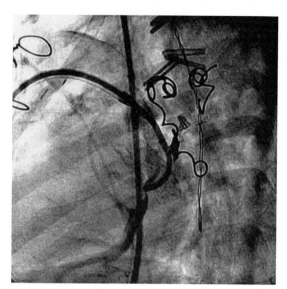

Fig. 32 Angiogram of side branch occlusion after stent placement

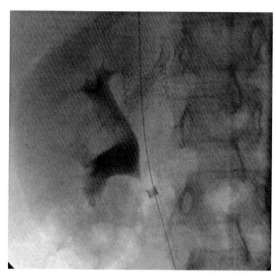

Fig. 31 Angiogram stent secured in SVC after free from Atrium

branches can be dilated and result in improved flow in the event of side branch compromise.

Fracture

Although more commonly seen when stents are placed in dynamic obstructions Fig. 33, this

Side Branch Compromise

Although the open stent is more than 90% free space, side branch compromise may occur if the orifice of the branch is straddled by the stent Fig. 32. This is more common when the branches take off at an acute angle and their opening is compromised by the expanded stent overlying the vessel proximally. Choice of length and positioning of the stent helps in avoiding this complication; however, this complication may be unavoidable and its consequence should be weighed against the gain in improvement of flow in the stented vessel. Simultaneous stenting can be performed in certain situations. In some stents (especially "open-celled" stents), the cells leading to side

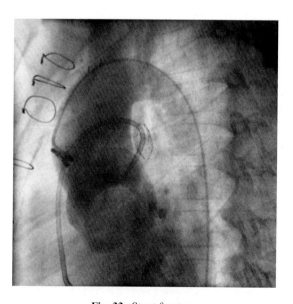

Fig. 33 Stent fracture

Table 8. Occlusion Devices for Atnal Septal Defects

	AMPLATZER®	Helex®	CardioSEAL®	STARFlex®
Manufacturer	AGA	GORE	NMT	NMT
Device design	Double mesh caps	Double spiral discs	Double umbrella.	Double umbrella
	Nonferromagnetic woven Nitinol (nickel–titanium alloy) mesh, two mushroom caps set end-to-end with 4-mm long connecting waist	Nonferromagnetic spiral Nitinol (nickel–titanium alloy) wire with attached Gor-Tex® (PTFE) fabric	Nonferromagnetic MP35n® (nickel–cobalt–chromium–molybdenum) alloy radial arms (4) with Dacron (polyester) fabric	Nonferromagnetic MP35n® (nickel–cobalt–chromium–molybdenum) alloy radial arms (4), spring (Nitinol) coil design, with Dacron (polyester) fabric
Centering method	Rigid, central disc	None	None	Microsprings adapt to variations in defect shape and septal morphology
Delivery method	6–12 Fr sheath, sequential disc deployment	9 Fr sheath, sequential disc deployment	10–11 Fr sheath, sequential umbrella deployment	10–14 Fr sheath, sequential umbrella deployment
Retrievability	Difficult after release	Limited data	Difficult after full deployment or release	
Conformability	Reported as not very conformable when defect is not round	Reported as very conformable	Occluder arms move independently from one another, enabling device to adjust to various septal morphologies	
FDA status	Approved for ASD and muscular VSD closure	Approved for ASD closure	Approved for VSD and Fontan fenestration closure	Pending

could also happen in stented pulmonary arteries especially if high-pressure balloons are used to place the stents. To avoid this, it is recommended that high inflation pressures be used for angioplasty prior to stent implantation allowing the stent to be positioned with relatively low pressures.

MRI Considerations

Many of the most common stents are made of 316 L stainless steel, which is a non-ferromagnetic material. In studies to date there appears to be no risk of movement or displacement of the stent during an MRI, even immediately after implantation. The stents may cause artifact due to distortion of the magnetic field.

Occlusion Devices

There is an ever-expanding list of vascular and septal occlusion devices available for use in the catheterization lab, a detailed discussion of which is beyond the scope of this manual. We will present some of the more common occlusion devices that are either FDA approved or available as part of FDA-approved clinical trials, Table 8. However, the Helex® device has not been used by the editors at the time of publication and therefore will not be discussed in detail.

Septal Occlusion

The purpose of this section is not to describe in detail which devices can or should be used where, but rather to provide a description of the general characteristics of the more commonly available devices.

CardioSEAL®/STARFlex®

These devices are self-expandable with a double-umbrella design. Each of the umbrellas has four spring-loaded arms which are flexible and attached to one another in the center

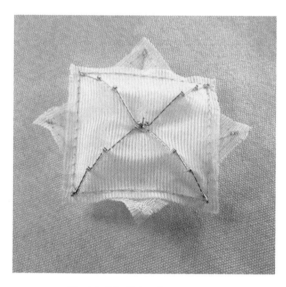

Fig. 34 NMT Cardioseal device

Fig. 34. This design allows arm separation when the septum is thick and arm overlap when the septum is thin, maintaining a low profile against the septum. The metal arms are covered with a woven Dacron fabric to promote early endothelialization.

ClamShell I: First-generation double-umbrella device available in 1989. The design was modified due to a high rate of arm fractures.

CardioSEAL®: Second generation; first used in 1996. This device is FDA approved for muscular VSDs and Fontan fenestration closure. Refer to chart in appendix for available sizes.

STARFlex®: Third generation. Major modifications include a flexible self-centering mechanism consisting of four flexible microsprings attached between the opposing umbrellas, a pin-pivoting delivery mechanism that allows pivoting of the device along the septal plane during delivery, and a smaller delivery profile. As of July, 2008 this device has not been FDA approved.

AMPLATZER®

The AMPLATZER devices are self-expandable, double-disc devices made from a Nitinol wire mesh. The two discs are linked together by a short connecting waist. The discs and waist are filled with polyester fabric that is secured to each disc by a polyester thread. There are several AMPLATZER® devices, each with a design specific for transcatheter closure of specific defects.

The AMPLATZER *Septal Occluder* (ASO) is FDA approved for transcatheter closure of secundum ASDs and fenestrations, and comes in sizes ranging from 4 mm to 38 mm. The two discs are linked together by a connecting waist, the diameter of which corresponds approximately to the stretched diameter of the ASD. The LA disc is larger than the RA disc (see chart in the Appendix).

The AMPLATZER *Multi-fenestrated "Cribriform" Septal Occluder* is currently available in four sizes (18 , 25, 30, and 35 mm). It has a similar design to the ASO described above but with a narrow central connecting stalk, and the LA and RA discs are each the same size. Ostensibly, it is designed for closure of multi-fenestrated ASDs such that the smaller central stalk allows placement through holes of relatively small size, but the more generous RA and LA discs allow coverage of a greater portion of septum, Fig. 35.

The AMPLATZER *Muscular VSD Occluder* is similar in design to the atrial septal occluder, except the central core is longer (7 mm) and the retention discs are the same diameter on both the RV and LV sides, with the diameter of the retention discs usually being 8 mm larger than the central core (except in the 4-mm device, where the difference is 5 mm).

The AMPLATZER *Ductal Occluder* is available in a variety of sizes (see chart in the

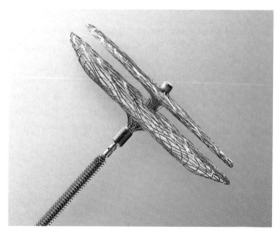

Fig. 35 AMPLATZER Multi-fenestrated septal occluder device

Appendix), with an aortic disc and narrower intraductal base. The device is placed transvenously. It is recommended that the size of the smaller end of the ductal occluder be 2 mm greater than the smallest dimension of the PDA.

The AMPLATZER *Vascular Plug* is available in a variety of sizes (see chart in the Appendix).

How to Load a Device

CAUTION: **Loading devices correctly is critically important, because a loading failure can result in device embolization. If you have any doubt that the device has been loaded properly, let the attending know. It is always easier to pull another system off the shelf than to try to recapture and remove a device.**

NMT Delivery System

The NMT delivery system consists of a long sheath and dilator, a delivery catheter/cable assembly, a "quick loader," and the device. The device is attached to the delivery catheter/cable using a pin-to-pin mechanism.

Loading a CardioSEAL/STARFlex® is a two-person task. One person holds the delivery catheter in the right hand, and the device in the other. The device should be oriented so that the pin at the end of the delivery cable and the pin on the device are side-by-side and are only overlapping by the length of the head of the pin. The second person will withdraw the delivery pin into the cupped sleeve at the end of the delivery cable. The pin of the device will then be trapped in the cupped sleeve, and cannot be released until the delivery pin is advanced out of the cupped sleeve.

Advancing and withdrawing the pin is accomplished by pushing or pulling the small black cylinder at the back end of the delivery cable. After the pin is withdrawn and the device has been attached, the relationship of the pin to the sleeve can be fixed by locking the black cylinder in position. Now that the device is on the delivery cable, it must be collapsed into the loader.

Person 1 will hold the buttoned thread of the distal arms of the device and pull as if pulling the device off the delivery cable. Person 2 will provide counter traction by pulling the delivery cable in the opposite direction. This will lengthen the entire system, and will collapse the distal arms of the device. While these arms are collapsed, Person 1 will slide the loader over these arms and then continue sliding until the entire device is collapsed into the loader. At this point, the buttoned thread can be cut away.

With the device attached to the cable, collapsed in the loader and free of the thread, it is almost ready to go. The only thing that remains is to flush the device and loader with some saline. Finally, Person 2 advances the blue catheter along the cable up to the loader and fixes the relationship by screwing down the black cylindrical vise. The purpose of the blue catheter is to add support to the delivery cable as the device is pushed up to its destination through the long sheath. When it is near the end of the long sheath the blue catheter can be withdrawn, exposing the cable within the sheath. The device is now ready for delivery.

AMPLATZER Delivery System

The AMPLATZER delivery system is similar for most of the devices and consists of a long sheath and dilator, a delivery cable, a loader, and the device. The device is attached to the delivery cable using a screw-in mechanism.

First, pass the delivery cable through the loader. Hold the cable in one hand and the device in the other. The device should be oriented so "male" and "female" parts of the screw-threaded release mechanism are lined up coaxially. Appose the two parts and start to attach the device by turning the cable a bit clockwise. When the cable and device can hold themselves together gently spin the device counterclockwise until it is fully screwed onto the end of the cable. You will feel a little resistance and then a "clunk" that indicates that the device is locked to the cable. Immerse the device, attached to the delivery cable, into a bath of flush solution. Holding the cable firmly with one hand and the loader firmly with the other, pull the cable and device back into the loader in one quick, smooth action. The device should collapse into the loader. Flush the loader. You are now ready to introduce the collapsed device into the long sheath for delivery.

Retrieving a Device

Not everything goes as smoothly as you would like in the catheterization lab, and if you spend enough time in the lab you *will* have to retrieve a device. In general, there are two types of device retrieval: retrieval of a device you have control of (delivery system still attached) and retrieval of a device that you don't have control of (malpositioned or embolized and not attached to a delivery system).

NMT Retrieval

CardioSEAL and STARFlex devices exist in one of four states in the body. They are either entirely within the delivery sheath, partially deployed ("LA" arms out, "RA" arms still in the sheath), fully deployed (all arms out, still attached to delivery cable), or released. Recapturing a partially deployed NMT device is straightforward. Depending on your situation you may either carefully pull on the delivery cable or slide the delivery sheath forward (or both). Either will easily recapture the "LA" arms, after which you may either reposition and redeploy or remove the device through the long sheath.

In contrast, after both sets of arms are delivered, things get somewhat more difficult. As discussed briefly above, the NMT devices cannot be pulled back into the usual delivery sheath in their entirety. They can, however, usually be pulled back partially (the pin and central body of the device typically may be pulled into the sheath, but the "RA" and "LA" arms will evert and overlap and not all come within the sheath). It is for this reason that we advocate for a 14 Fr short "safety sheath" in most situations because you can usually pull the device and delivery sheath combination out through a sheath of this size (and not lose access!).

To use this technique you can either place the 14 FR short sheath primarily and perform the intervention as planned through this, or before you place your long delivery sheath you can slide it through the short sheath and slide this all the way back to the hub of the long sheath. Depending on the patient's size, you may be able to leave the short sheath back and out of the body and only advance it over the long sheath if you need

to retrieve the device. Note that rarely when trying to retrieve a fully deployed NMT device into the long delivery sheath the device can dislodge from the delivery cable (and embolize). This may occur if the delivery cable has not been appropriately attached or locked onto the NMT device pin, so you should always exercise extreme care when loading your device! Finally, retrieving a released and either malpositioned or embolized NMT device is difficult and usually requires some combination of large long sheaths and snares.

Tips:

- When attempting retrieval of either a fully deployed or released NMT device, try to avoid recapture in the vicinity of cardiac or vascular structures that may become entrapped in the device/sheath (e.g., Eustachian valve, etc.), and *never* pull a device across a valve.
- When attempting retrieval of a fully deployes NMT device move to a secure position such as the IVC before aggressively trying to pull the device into the sheath therefore if the device becomes detatched from the cable it will be less likely to embolize.
- Always keep an eye on your ACT when resheathing and recapturing devices as thrombus may form on them and be embolized with manipulations.

AMPLATZER Retrieval

One of the chief benefits of **AMPLATZER** devices of essentially all types is that they are easily "resheathable" until released. After they are released, things again become a bit trickier. However, often the device can be snared or captured with a bioptome at the point where the delivery cable attaches and then can be fully retrieved into the delivery sheath (or more easily through a slightly larger sheath). Attempting to reattach the delivery cable to a released device by trying to screw them back together in situ is usually a waste of time because the cable is seldom in perfect alignment. Do not waste time snare the device and get it out of the body.

Vascular Occlusion

Coils

Cesare Gianturco, an Italian radiologist, first described the use of coiled spring "wooly tails" in 1975. Since that time, Gianturco-type coils have become commonplace in catheterization labs for occlusion of a variety of vascular (and other) structures. Coils come in a variety of shapes, sizes, and constituents, but share the common characteristic of a spring-like shaped metal coil, usually embedded with synthetic filaments that promote thrombosis Fig. 36. The most common coils in pediatric catheterization labs are made of steel or platinum. Steel coils are "MRI safe," but produce greater artifact than platinum coils. Steel coils also maintain greater radial force then platinum coils, but are somewhat more difficult to visualize on fluoroscopy. Recently, new non-ferromagnetic metal alloy coils were made available with similar characteristics to the steel coils. Ideal coil characteristics depend on the indication. Coil occlusion of PDAs

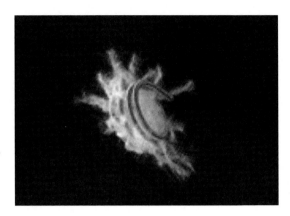

Fig. 36 A coil

is discussed in Section II. Most coils are delivered through shaped or end-hole catheters by carefully delivering the coil out of the catheter with a straight wire, or pulling back the catheter while holding the wire and coil in place. Detachable coils also exist and numerous technical modifications are possible including multiple coil and bioptome assisted delivery.

After the Case

Hemostasis

Holding the Groin

At the end of the case, you will usually have to give up your hard-fought vascular access. The most common means of achieving hemostasis in pediatric patients is still manual compression. There is actually a technique to pulling catheters and holding the groin. Groin hematomas are usually the result of poor holding technique in establishing and maintaining hemostasis, and occur relatively commonly, especially during a fellow's first month in the lab.

After the femoral renous sheath and arterial sheath or catheter are removed from their respective vessels, the most common mistake made is that pressure is placed directly on the puncture sites of the skin. The proper method is to place pressure at the puncture site of the vessel. The puncture site of the vessel is usually about a centimeter superior to the puncture site of the skin (see Figure 1). While applying pressure, one should be able to visualize the actual puncture sites to monitor for bleeding.

The next common mistake is to apply too much pressure to the site. Only apply enough pressure to prevent bleeding but not so much pressure that there is substantial venous congestion or loss of a pulse distally. This is particularly important in infants!

When people are first in the catheterization laboratory, they may be surprised at how long one must hold pressure onto a vessel to establish hemostasis. Holding pressure for durations of 30 minutes is not uncommon, and may be longer in a patient who has had a large sheath used or received systemic heparinization near the end of the case. Be patient when establishing hemostasis. It is better to wait a few more minutes than to let go, rebleed, and start the clock all over again.

Arterial Closure Devices (ACDs)

There are a number of mechanisms of assisted arteriotomy closure, other than just pushing, including Perclose®, Angio-Seal™, and Vaso-Seal® systems. Use of these is limited to larger children and adult patients because there are vessel-size requirements. Their possible benefits include decreased staff utilization time (you can sometimes hold compression for a long while), quicker room turnover (if you hold in the lab), and earlier time to patient ambulation and discharge. Studies in adults suggest probably no large difference in access complications in either diagnostic or interventional cases when compared to manual compression.

The most common ACDs at present are the Perclose and Angio-Seal devices. The Perclose system is a suture mediated closure mechanism, and there are no reaccess restrictions. The Angio-Seal device works by creating a mechanical seal by sandwiching the arteriotomy between a bio-absorbable anchor and a collagen sponge. Absorption is expected within 60–90 days. Reaccess prior to 90 days is possible, but it is recommended that access be obtained ∼1 cm proximal to the prior arteriotomy.

Sign Out

The cath lab is a busy place and between preparing your report, eating lunch, and preparing for your next case it is easy to forget to sign out your patient. Nevertheless, this is a vital part of

L. Bergersen et al. (eds.), *Congenital Heart Disease*,
DOI 10.1007/978-0-387-77292-9_4, © Springer Science+Business Media, LLC 2009

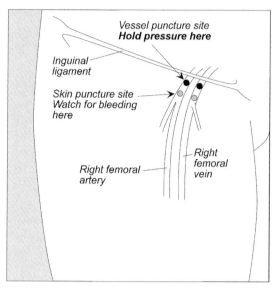

Fig. 1 Holding the groin

patient care. As soon as you have established hemostasis, your next step is to contact the ICU or ward and sign out to the team assuming care of the patient. The sign out should be brief and consist of a very concise history, reason for cath, access, preliminary hemodynamic and angiographic data, interventions done, and complications. You should mention any required therapies (heparin/antibiotics) or follow-up studies (CBC, lung scan, echo, etc.).

Talk to the Parents, Spouse, and/or Patient

Usually your attending will have talked to the parents or other family members right after the case. But you should know the patient and family from your precatheterization discussions. Stop in and see them. Be sure they know everything they should. Answer any new questions and make sure your patient is recovering well. Check the access sites for complications.

Writing a Report

This is *not* as bad as it will seem the first couple times. You will get the hang of this process. The goal is to concisely convey your (meaning both you and your attending's) hemodynamic and angiographic findings, as well as any interventions and their sequelae.

The most time-intensive process for new fellows is usually the translation of hemodynamic tracings to numeric values and interpreting the angiography. Both of these come easily, or more easily, with practice. The following are some hints to make your life easier:

1. Understand basic hemodynamics and the interpretation of basic intracardiac pressure recordings *before* you start the case.
2. Discuss the findings *during* the case with your attending.
3. Enter your hemodynamic values as soon as possible *after* the case because you may forget what you and the attending agreed upon, and the tracings may not be as good as you remember.

Mechanisms for generating catheterization reports will vary between institutions. In the most basic form, a note may be handwritten in the chart. However, more advanced options are now routinely used. Many catheterization reporting programs exist, some of which do much of your work for you, although you should always review any automated interpretations of tracings and calculations for accuracy. The best of these programs will generate a report for the chart and allow for future systematic inquiry. That is, it is important to report what you do, but it is equally important to be able to review your procedures to improve future outcomes.

Reports require a minimum amount of procedural detail, which should include:

Preprocedural Data

- Patient demographic data (name, medical record, date of birth, weight, BSA, hematocrit, etc.)
- Patient's diagnosis, clinical status, and indication for catheterization
- A succinct summary of prior medical, transcatheter, and surgical interventions

Procedural Data

- Patient condition during the procedure (include type of anesthesia/sedation, inotropes, FiO_2, etc.)
- Access sites
- Hemodynamic data (saturations and pressures) and interpretation
- Angiographic description (positive and negative findings) and total contrast load
- Interventions and their results (hemodynamic, angiographic or otherwise)
- Complications

Postprocedural Data

- Any recommended medications (anticoagulation, antibiotics, etc.)
- Any recommended studies (f/u lung scan, CXR, echo, etc)

The Next Day

It is not only a good idea to see your patient the day after their catheterization, but many attendings expect it. If your patient is under the primary care of another team, make sure they understand the postcatheterization care or follow-up that is required. Speak with the parents and check out your patient's access site(s). Do not rely on someone else (e.g., an intern) to know if your patient has a groin complication. This is your responsibility. Notify your attending if you have any questions or concerns.

Access Site Complications

You should *always* examine your patients after the procedure for signs or symptoms of access-related complications. Unfortunately, access site complications are not uncommon in cardiac catheterization procedures. Fortunately, most are not serious. Recognized risk factors include access site, smaller patient size, larger catheter/sheath size, interventional catheterization (as opposed to hemodynamic), the use of anticoagulation, and (particularly in adults) multiple comorbidities.

Access site complications can be generally divided into the following:

Minor Bleeding and Bruising

Minor bruising is common following central venous or arterial access and is not cause for concern. Patients and their parents should be told to expect this. Significant hematomas are usually the result of poor holding technique or multiple attempts at access. Large hematomas can be painful or hemodynamically compromising; more significant vascular injury should be considered and evaluated.

Major Bleeding

Localized bleeding from access sites after initial hemostasis is not uncommon and can be controlled by application of direct pressure and redressing. Risk factors include larger access catheters, arterial access, and anticoagulation. Forceful coughing or vomiting will often precipitate rebleeding. If patients are unable to detect the bleeding as in infants (diapers can hold a lot of blood) or intubated patients, significant blood loss can occur; therefore, careful monitoring is essential, particularly if patients are receiving anticoagulation or thrombolysis.

Retroperitoneal hemorrhage or hemothorax following femoral or subclavian access can be serious and life threatening. At Children's Hospital Boston, access sheaths are usually removed in the catheterization lab and patients are not transferred to recovery until hemostasis has been achieved. We routinely perform a final spot fluoroscopic examination in patients following subclavian access to assess for a possible hemothorax. Retroperitoneal bleeding may be asymptomatic and should be considered in any patient with femoral access and an unexplained hematocrit drop or excessive back discomfort, and should definitely be considered in any patient with unexplained hemodynamic instability. In larger children and adults, subcutaneous bleeding into the leg can also result in significant blood loss, but is usually more easily detected.

Vascular Trauma

Vascular occlusion can occur, particularly in infants and small children, when large access catheters are required. Meticulous attention to pulses and perfusion during and after hemostasis are critical. Acute venous occlusion can result in venous stasis and limb swelling. Acute arterial occlusion can result in anything from a mildly pale limb, to limb ischemia and loss. Therefore, while transient loss of pulse is relatively frequent in these patients, if pulses do not return within a short period of time, action is required. For patients with pulse loss but preserved perfusion, it is reasonable to start with unfractionated heparin. This should be at therapeutic levels with monitoring as appropriate. If this is unsuccessful or if perfusion is compromised, a TPA infusion should be initiated. Surgical or transcatheter thrombectomy is rarely required, but should not be delayed in situations where anticoagulation and thrombolysis are contraindicated or unsuccessful. The long-term consequences of vascular occlusion include limb length discrepancy, claudication, and inability to utilize that vessel for further catheterization.

Pseudoaneurysms occur and are usually manifest as a palpable pulsatile mass in the groin. Ultrasound will confirm the diagnosis. Small pseudoaneurysms may spontaneously thrombose. For more significant defects, surgical repair has been the historical gold standard, but direct compression and, more recently, ultrasound-guided thrombin injection may also be successful.

Arterial-venous (AV) fistulae are more common following femoral access but can occur anywhere. The clinical hallmark is palpable thrill or audible bruit. These probably result from incidental puncture of superficial vessels en route to the femoral artery or vein. When catheters are removed, a tract may develop between the two. Many AV fistulae spontaneously close, but patients will need to be followed to confirm this. Spontaneous resolution is probably less likely in patients on chronic anticoagulation. Surgical repair is the standard.

A Few Final Words of Advice

Getting Ready

- Do not forget to put on a mask before you scrub.
- Do not forget to take off your beeper before you put on your lead.
- Do not flush the balloon of the end-hole with saline.
- Make sure the table is set up before the attending is scrubbed. Look like you are doing something when the attending enters the room.

Access

- Do not stick the tech with the needle when getting lidocaine.
- Do not forget the lidocaine in the groin before you stick the groin.
- Do not inject the groin with heparin.
- Do not inject contrast through an angiocath without having the fluoroscopy on or being in an actual blood vessel.
- Do not forget to have a second wire available when you get access if the first wire becomes kinked or will not follow.
- Do not inject lidocaine instead of heparin after you get access.
- Do not forget to reassess your landmarks, if you get urine or spinalfluid. You are too deep!

During the Case

- Do not forget to put the balloon up on the wedge catheter before trying to get to the RV.
- Do not pull the wedge catheter out of the RV with the balloon inflated.
- Do not hand your attending a wedge catheter when they ask for a Berman.

- Do not leave the balloon up in the RVOT pending further instructions.
- Do not forget to tell the anesthesiologist when you are moving the cameras.
- Do not pull the wire out of a freshly dilated vessel before the angiogram is taken.
- Do not re-cross a freshly dilated area with wires.
- Do not put the stiff end of the wire out of the catheter and then step on cine.
- Do not lose wire position.
- Do not pull the wire out of the patient while trying to tidy up the table.
- Do not inject air.
- Do not forget to prep the balloons before they are inflated.
- Do not forget your night vision goggles to load the 0.014 invisible wires in the dark.
- If there are any problems it is definitely your fault. Just suck it up.
- Only the boss is allowed to throw catheters on the floor.

And Always Remember: If it did not work the first 10 times, why the *#$% is it going to work this time!?

At the End of the Case

- Do not forget to take off your lead before holding the groin.
- Do not make someone else hold the groin.
- Do not make giant bruises that require Urology to see the patient.
- Do not obstruct the vessels so much that there are no distal pulses, and the leg is purple.
- Do not forget to uncover the sites so you can see if there is any subcutaneous bleeding.

L. Bergersen et al. (eds.), *Congenital Heart Disease*,
DOI 10.1007/978-0-387-77292-9_5, © Springer Science+Business Media, LLC 2009

Part II
Specific Cases

The descriptions of cases and techniques presented in this manual are meant to serve as a general orientation to the subject matter for trainees in cardiology fellowships, and should not take priority over individual clinical and procedural decisions or simple common sense.

Institutional experience is provided when appropriate as well as pertinent references, and in some cases suggestions for additional reading. However, the references and resources are not meant to be an exhaustive review of the literature, and further reading on subject matter is encouraged, including original articles, reviews, and reports on other institutional experience and results.

Pulmonary Valve Dilation

Introduction

Isolated valvar pulmonary stenosis (PS) is a relatively common lesion, and one of the most straightforward cases you will perform. Typically, the pulmonary valve leaflets are thin and compliant with partially fused commissures, resulting in a dome-shaped valve structure with a narrowed central orifice. Dysplastic pulmonary valves are somewhat less common and differ in that they have irregularly thickened (myxomatous) valve leaflets, often with little, if any, commissural fusion. Leaflet mobility is variably reduced and the valve annulus may be small. The natural history studies provided a wealth of data about the course of this disease (1).

Natural History Data

Mild Pulmonary Valve Stenosis (RVp < 50% systemic; gradient 35–40 mmHg)

Patients with catheterization gradients of 35–40 mmHg (peak) had a normal hemodynamic response to exercise and had good long-term outcomes. When first diagnosed at less than 1 month of age, 29% progressed to moderate or severe obstruction; those that progressed did so in the first 6 months of life. Progression thereafter is very uncommon.

Moderate Pulmonary Valve Stenosis (RVp 50–75% systemic; gradient 40–60 mmHg)

These patients had excellent survival in the first and second natural history studies. By the end of the second natural history study (20 years later), most had surgery. They had decreased cardiac output and an abnormally increased RVEDp during exercise testing.

Severe Pulmonary Valve Stenosis (RVp > 75% systemic, gradient 60–70 mmHg)

Exercise testing in these patients showed irreversible changes in cardiac function if treatment was delayed. They had abnormal RVEDp at rest which increased with exercise. After valvotomy, they showed increased stroke volumes and decreased RVEDp.

Precatheterization Considerations and Case Planning

The work-up for isolated pulmonary valve stenosis is straightforward. Most patients will be subjectively asymptomatic. The physical exam should be consistent with isolated right ventricular outflow tract (RVOT) obstruction, with a systolic ejection murmur most notable at the left upper sternal border, often with an audible click and a systolic thrill. Most cases do not require extensive precatheterization ancillary studies. The CXR and ECG should be consistent with the referral diagnosis. From the echocardiogram, be sure you know the maximum instantaneous and mean Doppler gradients, pulmonary valve annulus measurement and qualitative RV function. Knowing the status of the atrial septum may prove useful because the patient with an atrial communication may be more stable with RVOT

L. Bergersen et al. (eds.), *Congenital Heart Disease*,
DOI 10.1007/978-0-387-77292-9_6, © Springer Science+Business Media, LLC 2009

occlusion. Most cases do not require either anesthesia or an ICU bed. Many institutions will elect to discharge the patient the same day if the procedure is uncomplicated.

As you plan for the case the important concepts and numbers for this case include:

- The peak-to-peak gradient from the RV to the MPA.
- The RVp/systemic pressure ratio.
- Know that increased right atrium *a* waves may indicate impaired RV compliance from severe or long-standing obstruction.
- Know that the RVEDp may be elevated with severe obstruction or with RV failure.

Procedure and Techniques

Generally these cases can be performed under conscious sedation. The femoral vein is cannulated with the appropriately sized sheath for the child's size to allow for adequate hemodynamics and angiography (5 Fr or 7 Fr). From the echo measurements of the valve diameter, you can get some estimation of what size balloon you will require. In the femoral artery, a 3–5 Fr pigtail catheter provides hemodynamic monitoring, although not all interventionalists will place an arterial catheter for this procedure.

After heparinization, routine hemodynamic measurements are obtained. The pulmonary valve usually can be crossed with a balloon end-hole (wedge) catheter, and then the gradient can be measured by pullback from the MPA. It is unusual for the catheter in this lesion to cause hemodynamic compromise by subtotal occlusion of the RVOT, but be prepared to take your balloon down.

Having established your gradient and excluded additional pathology, the end-hole catheter is removed and an angiographic catheter, such as a Berman, is then placed in the RV. The angiogram should be performed in cranially angulated PA and straight lateral projections with 1 cc/kg of contrast (maximum 15 cc for a 5 F and 22 cc for a 7 F Berman). The valve annulus can be measured best in the lateral projection in systole, measuring from hinge point to hinge point, and should be in fair agreement with the echo measurement.

After the angiogram is done, the pulmonary valve is crossed and an appropriate wire is placed in a lower lobe pulmonary artery. In this, as in all cases, there is nothing like good wire position! Take time to get it. The wire diameter depends on the type of balloon chosen. This is also the time to exchange the sheath if a larger one is needed for balloon dilation.

The usual balloon diameter is chosen to be about 120% of the pulmonary valve annulus. A 2-cm long balloon is used in young children to prevent damage to the right ventricular free wall. In older children and adults, a 3- to 4-cm long balloon can be used to facilitate appropriate balloon positioning.

In the older teenager or adult, the pulmonary valve annulus may be too large for single balloon dilation. In these patients, two balloons can be used together. The effective dilating size is not a single additive property but is actually an oval area encompassing both balloons with two triangular openings left between the two balloons when they are completely inflated, allowing some residual flow. A chart of the effective dilating size is provided in the appendix (2). If two balloons are used, two separate venous sheaths large enough for the balloons should be placed. Keep track of which balloon is which!

After the balloon is chosen and prepped, it is advanced over the wire and centered on the valve hinge points. The balloon is then inflated by hand and documented on cine. If the balloon is positioned well a waist should be seen in the middle portion of the balloon Fig 1. Further inflation of the balloon should result in complete obliteration of the waist. Complete obstruction of the RVOT is not always well tolerated and the balloon must be quickly deflated and passed into the PA or pulled back to the IVC (without damaging the tricuspid valve). The patient is allowed to recover from the dilation, and then the balloon is repositioned and inflated once more to ensure that there is no residual waist and that the balloon was positioned correctly. Be careful that the balloon is not too large (>130–140% of the valve annulus) or too far back, which can result in damage to the tricuspid valve apparatus. The dilating balloon is then removed, taking care to maintain wire position.

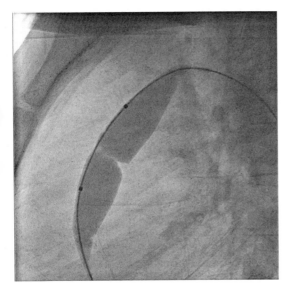

Fig. 1 Pulmonary valve dilation, adult

A catheter is then placed into the MPA and used to record a careful pullback gradient. Special care should be taken to determine if there is a subvalvar gradient contributing to any residual obstruction. Further angiograms may be required to redefine the anatomy. If obstruction persists at the valve, larger balloon sizes may need to be used, or the balloons may need better positioning for a better effect. We usually perform a final RV angiogram to qualitatively assess subvalvar obstruction and to exclude RVOT damage or tricuspid regurgitation.

Postcatheterization Care

This is usually uneventful. Routine access site care and a CXR may be performed.

Complications and Results

Complications are rare, especially serious complications. Perforation of the valve annulus or RVOT have been reported, although generally in association with oversized balloons (>140%

of the annulus diameter). Tricuspid valve injury is another serious but uncommon complication. Sustained arrhythmias are infrequent. In smaller patients, femoral vein occlusions have occurred. Bradycardia and desaturation are to be expected with the procedure, although they are typically very brief and well tolerated.

In a Children's Hospital Boston study, there was a significant reduction in transvalvular gradient from an average of 65 mmHg to 15 mmHg. Ninety-two percent of patients were left with gradients less than 25 mmHg. Calculated valve areas increased by 183% ± 80%. These results are comparable to other institutions. There is some evidence to suggest poorer results in patients with dysplastic valves (3).

Further studies on medium and late outcomes suggest a relatively low incidence of need for reintervention, and there is RV, tricuspid, and pulmonary valve annulus growth concurrent with somatic growth. Early pulmonary insufficiency is almost never a hemodynamic problem due to the low diastolic pressure of the pulmonary arteries. Progressive pulmonary insufficiency may occur over time, but the incidence and severity is currently unknown.

References

1. Nugent EW, Freedom RM, Nora JJ et al, Nadas AS. Clinical course in pulmonary stenosis. *Circulation* 1977;56:38–47.
2. Yeager SB. Balloon selection for double balloon valvotomy. *J Am Coll Cardiol* 1987;9:467–468.
3. Radtke W, Keane JF, Fellows KE et al. Percutaneous balloon valvotomy of congenital pulmonary artery stenosis using oversized balloons. *J Am Coll Cardiol* 1986;8:909–915.

Review Article

Gudausky TM, Beekman RH. Current options, and long-term results for interventional treatment of pulmonary valvar stenosis. *Cardiol Young* 2006;16: 418–427.

Critical Pulmonary Stenosis

Introduction

This is a bit more difficult than simple valvar PS as previously discussed. Patients with critical valvar PS are cyanotic at birth and require PGE maintenance of pulmonary blood flow. Right-sided hypoplasia is rarely a limiting factor in newborns with critical PS. The appearance of a dysplastic valve, by angiography or echocardiography, has not been found to predict dilation outcome in neonates (1).

Precatheterization Considerations and Case Planning

These patients are often in an intensive care unit (ICU) on PGE, but are otherwise seldom unstable, and often not intubated. Planning for the case requires assessment of individual patient risk. Anesthesia is usually required, because the babies will frequently develop apnea with sedation while receiving PGE. A full precatheterization echo evaluation of anatomy and function is vital, and attention should be paid to measurements of the PV annulus, RV size and function, TR and (as the severity approaches PA/IVS) tricuspid valve size. Don't give up your ICU bed when you bring the patient down because dynamic sub-PS and/or poor RV compliance may necessitate additional care.

Procedure and Techniques

Typically the RFV is entered and a 5 Fr sheath is placed. The umbilical vein can be used, but this is technically more difficult. Arterial access provides hemodynamic monitoring. After access is achieved, the patient is heparinized and hemodynamic measurements are made in the SVC, RA, and RV. An angiogram can be performed with a 5 Fr Berman in cranially angulated PA and lateral projections to determine the appearance and size of the PV and annulus. To place the Berman catheter in the RV apex, a Cook deflecting wire or a hand-bent stiff end of a guide wire may be necessary. In some cases when the RV is small an angiographic catheter will straddle the tricuspid valve and a hand injection through an end-hole catheter will be more appropriate. The annulus is measured as the distance between the hinge points of the valve in both views. There should be agreement between the echo and angiographic measurements. If there is substantial disagreement, one or both should be repeated.

The Berman is replaced with either a 5 Fr end-hole catheter, a shaped end-hole catheter, such as a 4-5 Fr Benson, Judkins Right, or cut Judkins left coronary catheter. If you are using a shaped catheter, it is usually necessary to shape the stiff end of a straight wire to guide the catheter across the TV. When the catheter is guided into the RV, the straight wire is removed, and a torque wire is advanced to the tip of the catheter. The catheter is then gently rotated clockwise to position the angled tip into the RVOT, pointing posterior toward the valve. The next part of the procedure must be done carefully. The floppy tip of the 0.014″ or 0.018″ or similar wire must be advanced across the pulmonary valve. You must be careful that the tip of the catheter is not embedded in the muscle because even the floppy tip of a wire can perforate the heart wall in the newborn as it exits the catheter.

Freedom of the tip of the catheter is confirmed with hand injections of a small amount of dye or the free movement of the wire tip out of

L. Bergersen et al. (eds.), *Congenital Heart Disease*,
DOI 10.1007/978-0-387-77292-9_7, © Springer Science+Business Media, LLC 2009

the catheter. Under fluoroscopic guidance, the floppy tip of the wire is gently tapped across the pulmonary valve until it finds the small opening and is advanced across the duct or into the distal LPA. Across the patent ductus arteriosus (PDA) and into the descending aoAa is the preferred and most stable wire position.

The final balloon diameter should be about 120% of the PV annulus. A smaller initial dilation can be considered such as a 2–4 mm, 1- to 2-cm long balloon which, after inflation, will allow easier delivery of the larger balloon. The final balloon is usually inflated twice. Dilation is usually well tolerated under this physiology. After the dilation, the balloon is removed, leaving the wire in position. Over the wire, a cut-off pigtail can be advanced, repeat hemodynamic measurements acquired, and follow-up angiography performed to assess for any injury/extravasation of contrast.

When the gradient is sufficiently reduced, a final set of hemodynamics is performed usually with an end hole catheter, paying attention to subvalvar gradients. While the patient is on PGE, the degree of success may be difficult to determine, as the RV pressure will still be near systemic in the setting of a large PDA. PGE may be discontinued in the lab following a technically successful dilation. The patient's saturation may continue to be low due to right-to-left atrial shunting related to impaired RV compliance.

Postcatheterization Care

Again, this is usually routine and unremarkable, although many of these patients will return to the ICU for observation while their PDA closes. A CXR is commonly performed.

Complications and Results

In a Children's Hospital Boston study, the valve was successfully crossed and dilated in 34/36 patients (94%). The RV/systemic pressure ratio fell from 150% to 83%; systemic oxygen saturation increased from 91% to 96%. Patients were often left with residual infundibular obstruction and mild cyanosis that resolves over time (weeks to months).

Pulmonary valve dilation in neonates is associated with a higher rate of complications than in older children and adolescents. Complications in a Children's Hospital Boston series occurred in 11/34 (31%) patients with serious events including death from sepsis and necrotizing enterocolitis, endocarditis, and RV perforation. Less serious events included transient arrhythmias, right bundle branch block, loss of pulse, and occlusion of the femoral vein (1).

Reference

1. Colli AM, Perry SB, Lock JE Balloon dilation of critical valvar pulmonary artery stenosis in the first month of life. *Catheter Cardiovasc Interv* 1995;34:23–28.

Review Article

Sommer RJ, Rhodes JF, Parness IA. Physiology of critical pulmonary valve obstruction in the neonate. *Catheter Cardiovasc Interv* 2000;50:$473–479.

Pulmonary Atresia with Intact Ventricular Septum (PA/IVS)

Introduction

Because some of the technical details of this procedure are different from those described in the section on critical PS, PA/IVS is described separately. Patients with short-segment (membrane-like) pulmonary atresia are cyanotic at birth and require PGE for maintenance of pulmonary blood flow. This is perhaps the most straightforward example of ductal-dependant pulmonary blood flow. Among those with PA/IVS there is a spectrum, ranging from those with relatively good-sized RV chambers to those with significant RV hypoplasia or RV-dependent coronary circulation (1). Some degree of tricuspid valve hypoplasia is the rule and generally follows RV hypoplasia. Nevertheless, many patients with PA/IVS can achieve a biventricular circulation, and often their first step toward this is a trip as a newborn to the catheterization lab for valve perforation and dilation.

Precatheterization Considerations and Case Planning

These patients are in the CICU and on PGE. Many, but not all, are intubated. Anesthesia support for the case is reccomended for this procedure because it requires precise intervention and the child is on PGE.

A full precatheterization echo evaluation of anatomy and function is vital, and attention should be paid to measurements of the pulmonary valve annulus, RV size and function, and tricuspid valve size and regurgitation. Even with very good technical results, sub-PS and/or poor RV compliance will usually necessitate postcatheterization ICU and/or surgical care.

Procedure and Techniques

Typically, the RFV is entered and a 4–5 Fr sheath is placed. Arterial access provides both hemodynamic monitoring and important angiography; usually a 3 F sheath is sufficient. After access is achieved, the patient is heparinized and limited hemodynamic measurements are made.

Next you need to access the RV. The precatheterization echocardiogram will give you some idea of how difficult this will be and what catheter you should use to try this. In those with a good-sized RV, a Berman catheter may fit in the RV enough such that none of the angiographic side-holes are in the RA. More frequently, the RV is too small and a simple balloon end-hole catheter will suffice. Alternatively, a shaped coronary catheter can be used for angiography and then positioned in the RVOT below the valve. To place any of these catheters in the RV, a Cook deflecting wire or a hand-bent stiff end of a guide wire is usually required. Once you've entered the RV, check the pressure. It is not uncommon to see RV pressures 1.5–2 times systemic.

Next, you need an angiogram. Because there is little outflow (except maybe TR) usually a hand injection will provide adequate anatomic detail. This initial angiogram is usually performed in straight PA and lateral projections and should demonstrate RV size, the RVOT, subvalvar region, and TR. You may even see a tiny jet of antegrade flow through the pulmonary valve that echo was unable to detect. Most

L. Bergersen et al. (eds.), *Congenital Heart Disease*,
DOI 10.1007/978-0-387-77292-9_8, © Springer Science+Business Media, LLC 2009

importantly, you should begin to identify the existence and extent of RV-coronary artery fistulae.

If additional views are needed they should be obtained. If there is evidence of RV-coronary artery fistulae selective coronary angiography should follow and the case should not proceed without detailed knowledge of the coronary supply. The criteria used for RV-dependant coronary circulation (RVDCC) are detailed in the section on coronary angiography (2). if you make this diagnosis your case is essentially done. You do *not* want to open the pulmonary valve. In contrast, if the patient does not have RVDCC the case really begins.

After your angiogram remove your angiographic catheter. What you need now is good anatomic understanding of the RVOT, pulmonary valve, and MPA. This is best achieved by hand injection from just above and below the pulmonary valve Fig. 1. Usually the best catheter to get you into the RVOT and just below the pulmonary valve is a JR coronary catheter, but use what works. To get the catheter there you will likely need a Cook deflecting wire or a hand-bent stiff end of a guide wire as discussed above. This can be tricky, because there is often little room to maneuver, but the bend in the wire should direct the catheter into the RV. After the catheter is through the tricuspid valve, gently rotate the catheter clockwise. You should be able to guide it gently into the RVOT. From there, gentle manipulation should allow you to seat it nicely under the valve. Carefully take the wire out now or before starting to manipulate into the RVOT (do not lose catheter position!. Perform a small hand injection. Once under the valve in RVOT.

At this point if there is any antegrade flow you should see it. If there is, you can try to very gently tap a 0.014″ or 0.018″ floppy wire across the valve. If this does not work after several attempts or if there is true atresia you will need to perforate the valve. Before doing so it is best to characterize the MPA, so take a cut-off pigail catheter, multipurpose, or another JR catheter and pass it though the PDA and into the MPA, just above the valve. A hand injection or power injection will show you the MPA anatomy; an angiographic catheter can be attached to the

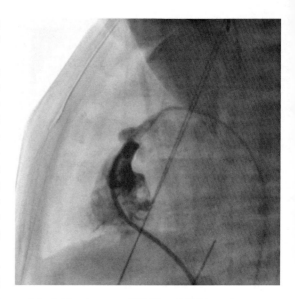

Fig. 1 Simultaneous RVOT and MPA angiogram

injector for future angiograms, thus guiding the perforation, and confirming proper wire position after perforation.

There are two common ways to perforate the valve. First, you can use the stiff end of a wire, usually slightly bent and with short, controlled quick movements try to pass it through the valve membrane. In the current era the more common technique is to use a commercially available radiofrequency (RF) wire through a coaxial catheter (0.035″ or 0.038″). These should fit through your JR catheter (or whatever catheter is positioned below the valve). Now, carefully align your RF wire in position. A common problem is for the RF wire to point straight (superiorly) out of the catheter, which if advanced any significant distance cannot only perforate the pulmonary valve but also the MPA as well. Thus, careful catheter and wire manipulations are needed with MPA angiograms as necessary.

The usual RF energy necessary is 5 Watts for 2 seconds. More than one attempt may be necessary. When the RF energy is applied, very gently apply forward pressure on the wire such that, if it is successful, it passes just beyond the valve. Again, angiograms in the MPA will confirm your position. Now slide the coaxial catheter over the RF wire, remove the wire, and run a 0.014″ wire through the catheter, across the valve and ideally through the PDA and into the dAo.

Initial dilation is often performed with a small (2–4 mm) balloon, inflated with a ~75% contrast solution until a waist disappears. This first inflation will create a defect large enough to allow your larger higher-profile balloon to pass through the valve. The final balloon should be about 120% the size of the pulmonary valve annulus Fig. 2. After the dilation, the balloon is removed, leaving the wire in position. Over the wire, a cut-off pigtail or end-hole catheter can be used to repeat hemodynamic measurements and perform angiography. Angiography is used to assess for injury/extravasation of contrast. Repeat dilation may be necessary. When successful, a final set of hemodynamics is performed, paying attention to subvalvar gradients.

As with critical PS, while the patient is on PGE, the degree of success may be difficult to determine, as the RV pressure will still be near systemic in the setting of a large PDA. Depending on the patient's likelihood of leaving the hospital without further intervention, PGE may be discontinued in the lab or in the ICU following a technically successful dilation. The patient's saturation will usually continue to be low to a variable degree due to right-to-left atrial shunting related to impaired RV compliance. If unacceptably low, the infant many require additional pulmonary blood flow (a shunt) until the RV starts to relax and accept blood. Pre-existing TR may improve if the valve is normal or may continue to plague the patient, making adequate antegrade RV flow difficult.

Postcatheterization Care

These patients return to the ICU for clinical observation as the ductus closes off PGE. A CXR and Hct are routinely obtained. Close observation, good groin care, and an ECG are necessary.

Complications and Results

Initial management at Children's Hospital Boston for newborns with PA/IVS is based on the presence or absence of RVDCC and rarely takes into account RV or tricuspid valve size. Those with RVDCC do not have RV decompression and undergo a BTS with the goal of single ventricle palliation. In a Children's Hospital Boston study 5-year actuarial survival for patients with RVDCC was 83%, with two early deaths presumably related to coronary ischemia (2,3).

In those with non-RVDCC, RV decompression is attempted based on the size of the RV and tricuspid valve, with or without a BTS. Subsequent decisions about their final physiology depends upon RV and tricuspid valve growth and function with patients undergoing either a single ventricle or "1-½ ventricle" palliation or ultimate biventricular repair. In terms of acute procedural complications, early mortality is usually related to unappreciated RVDCC and RV decompression as suggested above, and has not occurred in recent history. RVOT perforation can occur and may require pericardiocentesis or surgery.

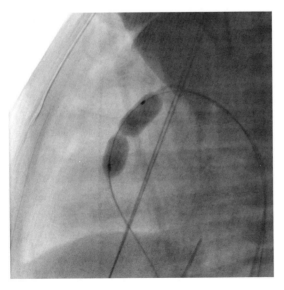

Fig. 2 Pulmonary valve dilation

References

1. Daubeney PE, Delaney DJ, Anderson, RH et al. Pulmonary atresia with intact ventricular septum range of morphology in a population-based study. *J Am Coll Cardiol* 2002;39:1670–1679.

2. Giglia TM, Mandell VS, Connor AR et al. Diagnosis and management of right ventricle–dependent coronary circulation in pulmonary atresia with intact ventricular septum. *Circulation* 1992;86:1516–1528.

3. Guleserian KJ, Armsby LB, Thiagarajan RR et al. Natural history of pulmonary atresia with intact ventricular septum and right ventricle-dependent coronary circulation managed by the single-ventricle approach. *Ann Thorac Surg* 2006;81:2250–2257.

Additional Readings

Agnoletti G, Piechaud JF, Bonhoeffer P et al. Perforation of the atretic pulmonary valve long-term follow-up. *J Am Coll Cardiol* 2003;41:1399–1403.

Humpl T, Soderberg B, McCrindle BW et al. Percutaneous balloon valvotomy in pulmonary atresia with intact ventricular septum impact on patient care. *Circulation* 2003;108:826–831

Aortic Valve Dilation

Introduction

In aortic stenosis the valve is most often bicuspid with a single fused commissure, either the intercoronary or right and noncoronary commissure. Less frequently, it is unicommissural, with an orifice at the left and noncoronary commissure (1). The course of left-sided disease is quite different from that of the right side. Again we well refer to the natural history study to review outcomes with aortic stenosis (2).

Natural History Data

Outcomes

- Endocarditis developed in 4% of patients.
- There was a 5% risk of sudden death.
- Most patients followed with even mild AS developed increasing obstruction over time.

Mild AS Gradient <25 mmHg (peak to peak systolic)

- Generally well tolerated.
- 21% risk of progression to need for surgery during 25-year follow-up.

Moderate AS Gradient 25–49 mmHg

- At this point intervention is probably not necessary.
- 41% of patients in this group ultimately received surgery in the Natural History Study.

Severe AS Gradient of >50 mmHg

- Gradient >80 mmHg is associated with a higher risk of sudden death and arrhythmia; intervention is recommended.
- 50 mmHg gradient is associated with an approximate 1% per patient-year risk of sudden death.
- In general, catheterization is indicated for a peak to peak systolic gradient of >50 mmHg.

Precatheterization Considerations and Case Planning

Precatheterization assessment is usually straightforward. Left-sided disease frequently is progressive, and this may not be the first time this patient has been to the lab. Know their history. Dilation as a newborn may mean occluded vessels. For all patients the consent discussion includes the risks and consequences of AR and the likelihood of re-intervention (catheterization or surgery). Discuss stroke. If you plan on using pacing during the case (see below), discuss this as well. The history, exam, CXR, and ECG should be in keeping with the diagnosis. Echo data should include maximum and mean gradients (the mean is often closer to what your peak gradient in the lab will be), degree of AR, LV size, and function and aortic valve annulus size. Be aware of known (and be prepared to rule out unknown) additional left-sided lesions (mitral stenosis and coarctation). The need for anesthesia will depend on many factors, but do not underestimate the effect of aortic obstruction on left atrial pressure. That said, an ICU bed is seldom necessary.

L. Bergersen et al. (eds.), *Congenital Heart Disease*,
DOI 10.1007/978-0-387-77292-9_9, © Springer Science+Business Media, LLC 2009

As you plan your case the most important number is the peak-to-peak systolic gradient between the LV and the aAo. Many factors affect the gradient, and must be considered. The most important of these is the transvalvar flow, because no flow means there will be no gradient. Ideally, the gradient and the transvalvar flow are measured at the same time. This can be done relatively quickly with thermodilution. If there is AR, most simple measurements of cardiac output will not take the regurgitant flow into account, so the gradient will actually overestimate the degree of obstruction. The mean LAp is usually normal. The LVEDp is generally in the high normal range due to LV hypertrophy and impaired compliance.

Procedure and Techniques

Aortic valve dilation outside of the neonatal period can usually be performed under conscious sedation. A femoral venous sheath is placed for routine hemodynamics +/– thermodilution and pacing if necessary. An arterial sheath is placed; in small children a 5 Fr sheath is placed, in older children a 6 or 7 Fr sheath is necessary. A pigtail catheter one size smaller than the sheath is placed through the arterial sheath. Heparin is given. Run the right side and obtain your output by Fick +/– thermodilution. In order to interpret simultaneous arterial recordings through the catheter and sheath correctly, it is necessary to make sure that the two transducers are balanced. The pigtail is moved to the aAo and the standing wave is calculated (standing wave = FA systolic pressure – aAo systolic pressure). An alternative in older children is to place another arterial catheter via the other femoral artery to record simultaneous LV and Ao pressures.

The pigtail is then placed in the LV. When the effective valve orifice is small, this can be quite difficult. Rather than use the standard looped pigtail to enter the ventricle, the soft end of a straight wire or torque wire through the straightened pigtail may be used to probe for the valve opening and then to guide the pigtail into the LV. Alterations of pigtail positioning or other shaped catheters may be necessary to get the correct angle to access the orifice of the stenotic valve (usually aiming leftward and posteriorly).

NOTE: *The open commissure is usually between the left and non coronary cusp. When you have the wire in the LV (be sure it is not in a coronary), feed wire into the LV apex before advancing the pigtail to avoid ensnaring the catheter in the mitral valve. The gradient can determined by calculating the (LV pressure – FA pressure) + the standing wave. (e.g., if the LV is 150, the FA is 90, and the standing wave is 8, then the PSEG is 68).*

In most cases, the catheter is pulled back to the aAo while recording the gradient by direct pullback. It is usually a good idea to record the ascending aortic pressure before entering the LV. If it has been particularly difficult to cross the valve, you may not want to pull back into the ascending aorta prior to dilation. With a pigtail in the LV, an angiogram is performed in the long axial oblique and RAO projections. This view allows a good image of the AoV leaflets. The annulus diameter is measured at the hinge points of the leaflets. The pigtail is placed in the aAo to perform an aortogram (generally in the same projections; you do not want to move the cameras and lose your markers for dilation). This is done to assess the amount of aortic regurgitation at baseline.

A simple alternative to this exists if there is an atrial defect (ASD or PFO) by which a catheter (end-hole or Berman) is placed antegrade (across the atrial septum and mitral valve) into the LV. Simultaneous LV and aAo pressures in this manner provide simultaneous pressures and the most precise gradient measurments. Angiography can also performed antegrade in the LV with a Berman Catheter.

If the patient's gradient and the degree of AR indicate the need for dilation, the pigtail is advanced over a wire into the LV apex. A stiff wire is placed in the LV. The end is hand-curved so that there is a broad curve of wire in the LV with a second curve in the arch such that the stiff part of the wire is across the annulus. When the aortic valve orifice is posterior, between the left and noncoronary cusps, the wire may course posteriorly and through the MV chordae. If the balloon is inflated with the wire in this position, it will damage the anterior MV leaflet. If lateral fluoroscopy demonstrates a wire course clear of the mitral valve, the balloon can be advanced over the wire otherwise alternative wire position should be obtained.

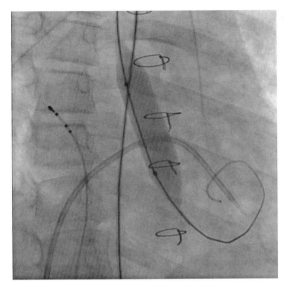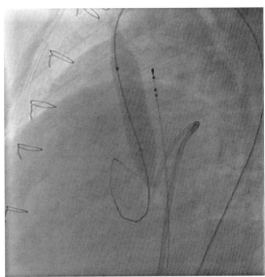

Fig. 1 Aortic valve balloon valvotomy

In a young child, use a 2-cm length balloon and for older children and adults use a 4-cm length balloon. The initial balloon size chosen should be 80–90% of the annulus size. The degree of aortic damage and regurgitation increases as the balloon-to-annulus ratio increases, very significantly so at 125%. The balloon is advanced until a little more than half of the balloon is below the valve. It should not be advanced further into the LV and then withdrawn into the aAo, as this tightens the catheter curve in the Ao and increases the likelihood that the balloon will be ejected with ventricular contraction.

Usually a lower contrast/saline ratio is used in balloons for aortic valve dilations with the goal of being able to adequately see the balloon (and waist), but also able to deflate the balloon quickly (contrast is much more viscous than saline or blood). The balloon is inflated until the waist is gone Fig 1. In older children and adults it may be necessary to rapidly pace from the venous side to maintain more stable balloon position during inflation. When the balloon is deflated, it is pulled to the dAo, then removed from the body when fully deflated.

After the dilation, the gradient is measured again and an angiogram is repeated to assess AR. If the gradient has not been adequately reduced and there is no change in AR, the next balloon size is inserted, or the same-size balloon is overinflated.

We try not to exceed the annular diameter with our largest balloon. If the gradient reduction is satisfactory, or if there is an increase in the degree of AR, the dilations are stopped. After dilation, a full set of hemodynamics is performed, including cardiac output.

Postcatheterization Care

These cases frequently call for somewhat large sheath sizes in the femoral arteries. Exceptional care should be given to perfect hemostasis without inducing occlusion. An arteriotomy closure device may be used in older children and adults to facilitate hemostasis. A CXR is usually performed.

Complications and Results

In most cases a gradient reduction of at least 50% can be achieved. In early reports, Children's Hospital Boston reported significant regurgitation (26%) with valve balloon ratios greater than 1.0 compared to ratios less than 1.0 (11%) but with no difference in gradient reduction achieved (3). Later, midterm results were reported and the 8-year survival was 95% with 50% of patients free from re-intervention (4). Similar results have been reported from other institutions (5). In the late 1990 s, the experience with repeat balloon dilation was published and patients who underwent initial dilation as a neonate were more likely to undergo re-intervention. The incidence of AR in this population of patients requiring repeat dilation was higher and graded as at least moderate in 24% after the second procedure (6).

References

1. Roberts WC. The structure of the aortic valve in clinically isolated aortic stenosis: an autopsy study of 162 patients over 15 years of age. *Circulation* 1970;42:91–97.

2. Wagner HR, Ellison RC, Keane JF et al. Clinical course in aortic stenosis. *Circulation* 1977;56:147–156.

3. Sholler GF, Keane JF, Perry SB et al. Balloon dilation of congenital aortic valve stenosis. *Circulation* 1988;78:351–360.

4. Moore P, Egito E, Mowrey H et al. Midterm results of balloon dilation of congenital aortic stenosis: predictors of success. *J Am Coll Cardiol* 1996;27:1257–1263.

5. Pedra CA, Sidhu R, McCrindle BW et al. Outcomes after balloon dilation of congenital aortic stenosis in children and adolescents. *Cardiol Young* 2004;14:315–320.

6. Satou GM, Perry SB, Lock JE et al. Repeat balloon dilation of congenital valvar aortic stenosis: immediate results and midterm outcome. *Cathet Cardiovasc Intervent* 1999;47:47–51.

Critical Aortic Stenosis

Introduction

The aortic valve in these patients is most often myxomatous and bicuspid with a single, fused commissure and an eccentrically placed orifice, or unicuspid (dome-shaped). The valve annulus may be small for age, but there is evidence that following dilation even quite small annuli may grow to a normal or near normal dimension (1). Myxomatous valves may mature, as Myxomatous pulmonary valves. Because there is a spectrum to left-sided obstructive lesions, often the first decision in many of these patients is whether they should have a valvotomy or a staged one-ventricle repair.

Precatheterization Considerations and Case Planning

These patients are generally quite ill, on PGE and intubated when they are brought for catheterization. The precatheterization assessment is similar to that of AS (as above), but with close attention to other left-sided structures as well as LV size and function. A low aortic valve gradient in the setting of ventricular dysfunction does not mean there is no important obstruction. Knowing the valve annulus is critical. Preprocedural AR is very unusual.

In the lab the two most important pieces of information are the mixed venous saturation and the aortic valve gradient as this sets the stage for the rest of the case. Be sure to identify any additional left-sided lesions such as mitral valve stenosis, subaortic stenosis, or coarctation.

Procedure and Techniques

The dilation can be approached from either a retrograde or antegrade direction. Remember that critical AS is a case of millimeters—so you need to be meticulous.

Retrograde Approach

This is the more common approach at Children's Hospital Boston since the production of low-profile balloons. Often the umbilical artery and vein already have been cannulated, and may be the only sources of access and monitoring for the patient. Generally, a 3–4 Fr sheath is placed in the femoral artery and a 4 or 5 Fr sheath in the femoral vein. Alternatively, other institutions have reported using a surgical cutdown on the right common carotid artery for a direct route to the aortic valve, although this is not practiced at most institutions. When arterial access is established, the infant is heparinized.

The LV-to-Ao gradient can be simultaneously recorded by passing a Berman antegrade across the PFO to the LV, with a pigtail catheter in the aAo. Next, angiograms need to be taken of the LV through the Berman, and in the aAo through the pigtail catheter. The angiograms should clearly demonstrate the annulus size, valve anatomy, degree of AR, and LV anatomy, size, and function. The next step is to cross the AoV with the floppy end of a 0.014″ or 0.018″ torque (or similar) wire via a straightened pigtail. Often the left-non commissure is patent and the wire can be advanced by tapping the wire leftward and posterior. The angiographic flow jet on the LV angiogram can be

L. Bergersen et al. (eds.), *Congenital Heart Disease*,
DOI 10.1007/978-0-387-77292-9_10, © Springer Science+Business Media, LLC 2009

used as a guide for crossing through a true orifice of the valve.

After the wire crosses the valve and enough wire is advanced to loop in the apex, the pigtail is guided into the LV. The 0.018″ torque wire is traded for a preshaped wire with the stiff-shaped part of the mandril matching the curve of the aortic arch. This prevents damage to the aortic arch wall when the balloon is delivered and subsequently inflated. The wire is placed in the LV apex along the septum, anterior to the MV chordae. The initial balloon is chosen to be 80–90% of the aortic valve annulus and usually 2 cm long. The balloon is fully inflated by hand across the valve, deflated, and then immediately pulled to the dAo.

The gradient, LVEDp, and mixed venous oxygen saturation are measured, and an ascending aortogram is performed to evaluate AR. Successful dilations are indicated by a decrease in gradient, a decrease in left atrial pressure, or both. Often the function is poor and the gradient is low even at the baseline. Success is declared when the gradient is less than 30 mmHg, or the largest reasonable balloon has been inflated across the valve. If success has not been achieved, and there is no increase in AR, then repeat dilation can be performed. The same size balloon is inflated at higher pressure, or sized up to the next available size. Low-profile, highly compliant balloons may achieve effective diameters much larger than the nominal. Therefore, measure the diameter of the balloon after dilations rather than rely on the number on the shaft.

Antegrade Approach

This approach is easier if the LV is somewhat dilated. The initial hemodynamics and angiography are performed as above. After the LV angiogram is performed, a 5 Fr long sheath is shaped to the course through the PFO, LA, and LV. The sheath is advanced over a 5 Fr balloon-tipped end-hole catheter to the LV apex. If the sheath induces significant MR, the sheath is removed and reformed. After the sheath is in the LV apex, the end-hole catheter is advanced across the AoV and into the dAo. Often a deflectable wire, or shaped stiff-end of a straight wire, will be necessary to make the turn at the apex. With

the catheter tip well into the dAo, a wire is shaped with an LV apical and aortic arch bend. After the wire is in position, the end-hole catheter is removed and the balloon is advanced. Balloon choices are made the same way as in the retrograde approach. The postdilation pressures and gradient can be measured through the catheter in the aAo and sheath in the LV.

Postcatheterization Care

There is a significant risk of femoral vessel loss after this procedure. You have to do what is necessary during the procedure, but you should be as gentle as possible in holding the groin afterward. Constantly feel for pulses. Heparin should be considered early for legs showing signs of compromised perfusion. Otherwise, we routinely obtain postcatheterization CXR and echocardiogram. These children usually recover in the ICU while the PGE is discontinued. It is not unusual to see small increases in residual echo gradient estimates as ventricular function improves.

Complications and Results

Our experience with neonatal patients with critical aortic stenosis treated by aortic valvotomy are reported in two manuscripts (1,2). Most recently, in a group including 113 patients, 78 were performed retrograde and 35 antegrade. Average immediate gradient reduction was 54%. We have observed a reduction in mortality in recent eras: mortality was 22% in the period 1985–1993 and 4% in the period 1994–2002. Life-threatening complications have included endocarditis, valve or heart perforation, and cardiac arrest.

Among 91 survivors with a biventricular circulation, freedom from moderate to severe AR was 65% at 5 years. Freedom from re-intervention on the LVOT was 65% at one year and 48% at 5 years. Re-intervention was associated with younger age, higher pre- and postaortic valve gradients, and larger balloon-to-annulus diameter ratios. Some patients have required surgery; freedom from aortic valve replacement was 84% at 5 years.

References

1. McElhinney DB, Lock JE, Keane JF et al. Left heart growth, function, and reintervention after balloon aortic valvuloplasty for neonatal aortic stenosis. *Circulation* 2005;111:451–458.

2. Egito ES, Moore P, O'Sullivan J et al. Tranvascular balloon dilation for neonatal critical aortic stenosis: early and midterm results. *J Am Coll Cardiol* 1997;29:442–447.

Mitral Valve Dilation

Introduction

Mitral valve (MV) dilation was first developed for adults and adolescents with rheumatic MV disease. It was then extended to children with congenital mitral stenosis (MS). Congenital MS is a morphologically heterogeneous lesion that generally affects both the valvar and subvalvar tension apparatus of the MV. Subtypes of congenital MS include "typical" congenital MS (which consists of thickened leaflets, short or absent chordae tendineae, obliteration of interchordal spaces, and two separate but often closely spaced papillary muscles), supravalvar mitral ring, parachute MV, and double-orifice MV. In many patients, there are features of multiple MS subtypes. Commonly associated lesions include other left heart obstructive anomalies (e.g., coarctation of the aorta, valvar or subvalvar aortic stenosis) and/or a VSD.

The clinical manifestations of congenital mitral stenosis vary with the degree of obstruction to LV inflow, the presence and type of associated lesions, and growth rate of the infant. In utero, LV inflow obstruction is of no hemodynamic consequence, because infants with mitral atresia will otherwise develop normally. Postnatally, patients with congenital MS typically present beyond the neonatal period with a history of antecedent pulmonary infection, poor weight gain, irritability, diaphoresis, tachypnea, and chronic cough.

Mitral valve dilation for congenital mitral stenosis is commonly used as a palliative procedure, to delay the need for surgical valve replacement/repair until the patient has grown to a larger size, in an attempt to decrease the number of future revisions for growth. It may also be used for treating MS after AVC repair or other mitral valve surgery. It is much more successful for rheumatic heart disease in preventing the need for surgery, as a means of therapy.

Precatheterization Considerations and Case Planning

Precatheterization assessment should be consistent with the diagnosis. Clinical symptoms associated with poor outcome include signs of low cardiac output and right heart failure. On exam, pulses and perfusion are diminished, and the RV impulse may be increased from pulmonary hypertension. In most cases, the first heart sound is diminished because the mitral leaflets are generally inflexible and immobile. This finding is in sharp contrast to rheumatic MV disease. The second heart sound varies from widely split to narrowly split with an accentuated P2 component when pulmonary hypertension is present. Third or fourth heart sounds may be present.

Careful echocardiographic evaluation is necessary to detect the exact anatomy of the MV disease, and to determine whether a supravalvar mitral ring is present. In patients with MS due primarily to a supravalvar mitral ring, balloon dilation is not effective. Three-dimensional echocardiography has proven helpful in defining the anatomy of the inflow orifice. The severity of MS is determined by a combination of factors, including clinical status, symptoms, and the LA-LV pressure gradient. Doppler echocardiography is used to estimate a maximum instantaneous gradient and a mean gradient. Severity is often graded as follows, although it is more informative simply to state the maximum and mean gradients:

L. Bergersen et al. (eds.), *Congenital Heart Disease*,
DOI 10.1007/978-0-387-77292-9_11, © Springer Science+Business Media, LLC 2009

- "Mild" stenosis 8–10 mmHg maximum gradient.
- "Moderate" stenosis 11–15 mmHg maximum gradient.
- "Severe" stenosis >15 mmHg maximum gradient.

MV dilation in older children may be performed under conscious sedation, although general anesthesia with positive pressure ventilation is quite appropriate, because there is a real risk of pulmonary edema with balloon dilation of the mitral valve. A postcatheterization ICU bed may be reserved in case of complications, but it not usually necessary in the absence of significant associated high-risk factors. Particularly in young or very sick children, a dopamine infusion may be readied and often started prophylactically before the interventional portion of the case.

Procedure and Techniques

Femoral arterial and venous access is obtained and secured with sheaths. The arterial catheter is used for pressure measurement, blood sampling, and angiography. Also, typically a pigtail catheter of sufficient length and caliber to perform LV angiograms is used. Femoral venous access is secured with a sheath of sufficient size to accept the appropriate balloon end-hole catheter for hemodynamic evaluation. After access is established, the patient is heparinized. A full hemodynamic evaluation is performed, including simultaneous measurement of LV and PA wedge pressures.

If a PFO or ASD is not present, a Brockenbrough puncture is necessary and a transseptal sheath of adequate size to deliver the dilating balloon(s) is advanced into the LA. Simultaneous measurement of LA and LV pressures is performed, and the mean transmitral gradient is calculated. The interatrial septum is often thick and bowed to the right, particularly in patients with long-standing LA hypertension. Thus, transseptal puncture may be more difficult than usual, and it may be necessary to dilate the septal puncture site with a 4–6 mm balloon in order to advance the long sheath into the LA.

After the hemodynamic evaluation, an LV angiogram is performed through the pigtail catheter

in the LV in the RAO projection to outline the MV annulus and to evaluate MR. After the angiogram, depending on the size of the patient a 5 Fr or 7 Fr end-hole catheter is passed antegrade from the LA to the LV and advanced to the apex, usually with the aid of a shaped wire. It is important to ensure that the balloon is inflated to avoid entering the LV through a secondary orifice or an interchordal space. A 0.018″ or 0.035″ wire is advanced through the end-hole catheter and left in the apex of the LV. The end-hole catheter is exchanged over the wire for the first dilating balloon.

In contrast to earlier practices, in which balloon size was selected on the basis of the annulus diameter, we now select the initial balloon primarily on the basis of patient size. The reason for this is that the mitral annulus is usually large in patients with mitral stenosis and consequent LA dilation, and generally does not reflect the size of the inflow orifice; moreover, unlike semilunar valve dilations, trauma to the annulus leaflet junction is probably an uncommon mechanism of dilation-related mitral regurgitation. You will discuss this with your attending, but a general guide to initial balloon sizing (1) is to select a balloon diameter of:

- 8 mm for BSA $\leq 0.4\,M^2$.
- 10 mm for BSA ~ 0.4–$0.8\,M^2$.
- 12 mm for BSA ~ 0.9–$1.2\,M^2$.
- 15 mm for BSA $\geq 1.2\,M^2$.

The balloon is inflated by hand, and then deflated immediately and withdrawn to the LA to allow for improved LV inflow during complete balloon deflation Fig 1. The balloon is removed, and repeat hemodynamic evaluation is performed along with angiography to evaluate for MR. If there is not adequate relief of MS, progressively larger balloons are used until satisfactory reduction in the gradient is achieved or mitral regurgitation is increased. Balloon size is also varied by modulation of the inflation pressure. Thus, each balloon is generally inflated twice, first at low pressure (2–4 atm), yielding an effective diameter less than the stated balloon size, and then again at a higher pressure, allowing relatively fine gradation of inflation diameter. Most patients undergo at least three or four dilations before a satisfactory result is achieved. At the end of the case,

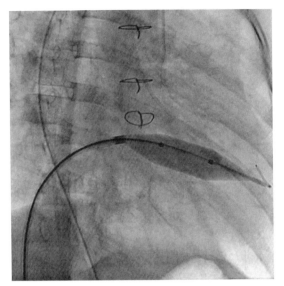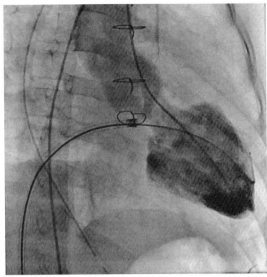

Fig. 1 Mitral valve balloon valvotomy

a full set of hemodynamics is performed with an estimation of right-to-left shunt if the atrial septum is dilated. Angiography in the LV should be performed at the end of the case without any wires across the MV to assess the true degree of MR after all dilations are completed.

Postcatheterization Care

Decisions regarding extubation, maintenance of the dopamine infusion, admission to the CICU, and so on, depend on the circumstances of the particular case. Anticoagulation/antiplatelet therapy is typically not required. Follow-up evaluation should include a repeat echocardiogram later in the day or the next morning.

Complications and Results

In older children and adults most of the complications of the procedure are short-lived and self-limited, including transient hypotension and arrhythmias, cardiac perforation without tamponade, increased mitral regurgitation, and small persistent atrial shunting. Infants are much more unstable going into the catheterization, and they have greater instability during the procedure, including profound bradycardia, heart block, and hypotension progressing to cardiac arrest.

Among 70 patients undergoing balloon dilation for congenital MS at Children's Hospital Boston between 1985 and 2003, the peak and mean catheterization-derived MS gradients decreased by a median of 33% and 38%, respectively. Maximum and mean Doppler gradients after MV dilation were 20% and 40% lower (median), respectively, than prior to intervention. Calculated effective MV orifice area increased by $74 \pm 69\%$, from 0.9 ± 0.3 to $1.6 \pm 0.7\,\mathrm{cm^2/m^2}$. Moderate or severe MR developed in 28% of patients after balloon dilation. Among patients who underwent MV dilation, freedom from failure of biventricular repair or MV replacement was 79% at 1 month and 55% at 5 yrs, with worse outcome in younger patients and those who developed significant postdilation MR. Hospital mortality among these 70 patients who underwent mitral valve dilation for congenital MS at Children's Hospital Boston was <5%.

Reference

1. McElhinney DB, Sherwood MC, Keane JF et al. Current management of severe congenital mitral stenosis outcomes of transcatheter and surgical therapy in 108 infants and children. *Circulation* 2005;112:707–714.

Pulmonary Angioplasty

Introduction

While the basic principles of angioplasty are the same for different vessels in the body (pulmonary artery, systemic vein, systemic artery, etc.) the procedures do have important differences with regard to the technique and choice of balloons. The goal of angioplasty is to create a controlled tear in a vessel wall so that the vessel can heal in the newly created diameter following relief of the stenosis. The ability of a balloon to tear a vessel is determined by the properties of both the vessel being dilated and the balloon being used. Therefore, the balloon chosen will depend on the site requiring dilation and individual balloon characteristics (see the Appendix). The most common sites requiring balloon angioplasty in congenital cardiac catheterization are the pulmonary arteries. Thus this section will focus on details pertinent to pulmonary angioplasty, but the concepts can be applied to other obstructed vessels.

The most common indication for balloon angioplasty of peripheral pulmonary artery stenosis is an angiographic narrowing in a peripheral pulmonary artery (single or multiple) with significant reduction in lumen causing:

1. Marked decrease in flow to the affected lung as assessed by radionuclide scan, or...
2. Significant pressure gradient across the area of stenosis, resulting in near-systemic or higher RV pressure and/or hypertension in unaffected portions of the pulmonary vascular bed (presumably secondary to increased flow), or...
3. Symptoms (fatigue, exercise intolerance, limitation of life style).

Pulmonary artery dilation can be performed at any age; however, elective procedures are frequently performed between the ages of 1 and 4 years as it is less hazardous than procedures done in infancy and may produce better results than procedures done later on in childhood or adulthood. If stenting is necessary, the patient is usually large enough at this age (10–20 kg) to allow placement of a stent that will be adequate to accommodate future lung development, vessel enlargement, and increased flow. Patients with TOF/PA or severe PS with hypoplastic pulmonary arteries may benefit from restoration of distal flow by relieving multiple PA stenoses in the first year of life.

Tetralogy of Fallot with or without pulmonary atresia is the most common diagnosis requiring pulmonary angioplasty. Other patients requiring PA angioplasty include surgically induced proximal branch stenosis in patients with other congenital heart disease, and isolated peripheral pulmonary stenosis sometimes associated with syndromes such as Alagille's or Williams.

Precatheterization Considerations and Case Planning

The precatheterization assessment of these patients can be quite involved because they will frequently have had numerous previous interventions.

- Always know the clinical status of your patient.
- A formal exercise study may be helpful.
- Pay attention on your exam for evidence of RVOTO, PR, and signs of RV failure.

L. Bergersen et al. (eds.), *Congenital Heart Disease*,
DOI 10.1007/978-0-387-77292-9_12, © Springer Science+Business Media, LLC 2009

- Continuous murmurs may suggest residual aorto-pulmonary collaterals.
- Include in your assessment a history of previous surgical procedures and catheter interventions including previous access issues and angioplasty sites, balloon sizes, inflation pressures, and results including change in lung scans.
- An echocardiogram should include estimation of RV pressure and function, site and severity of proximal pulmonary stenosis, and residual cardiac defects if present.
- In individual cases, MRI may add information about anatomy, RV function, PR fraction, and occasionally regional distribution of APC supply.
- A lung scan will help to determine the distribution of pulmonary blood flow.
- In cases expected to be long or complicated, anesthesia and/or a postcatheterization ICU bed may be required. Patients with Williams syndrome may be at higher risk from the procedure, due to the associated supravalvar aortic stenosis and coronary involvement in some of these patients Fig. 1. Proceed with caution during initiation of sedation/anesthesia. Creation of an ASD prior to angioplasty in such patients may make the patient more stable.

Procedure and Techniques

Arterial and venous access is obtained with appropriate sheaths. Attention should be paid to prior catheterization and dilation attempts. Optimal distal catheter or long sheath position to reach a difficult branch may require access from some place other than the groin (RIJV or LSCV). Single PA dilations or uncomplicated dilation procedures may be done with a short sheath by delivering balloons over a wire. However, in cases of multiple dilations a long sheath helps to secure stable position, allows rapid exchange of catheters and balloons, provides a route for efficient angiography, and in the case of a PA trauma, ensures reliable and rapid delivery of balloons, stents, or coils if necessary.

Many long sheaths require a separate hemostatic side-arm adapter, so after the long sheath dilator is removed, a side arm is mounted onto the wire (either with a short dilator or placed over the next catheter to be passed through the sheath). After flushing, contrast should be attached to the side arm of the sheath with a 10- or 20-cc syringe and refilled as necessary for adequate hand injection angiograms through the sheath. As an alternative to a long sheath, a second venous line may be placed to perform angiography. If you use a long sheath, be sure to be meticulous about flushing it and pay attention to anticoagulation because clots can and will easily form in these long tubes.

Hemodynamics

The procedure begins with a thorough hemodynamic assessment. A precise and accurate measurement of RV-to-Ao pressure ratio is important. Balancing the transducers with the catheters in these positions verifies the accuracy of the ratio. In rare cases of severe bilateral pulmonary stenosis with supra-systemic RV pressure and/or severe RV dysfunction, one should determine patency of the foramen ovale, because an atrial defect can support cardiac output during dilations. Rarely, a transseptal puncture with balloon dilation of the atrial septum may be planned as part of the

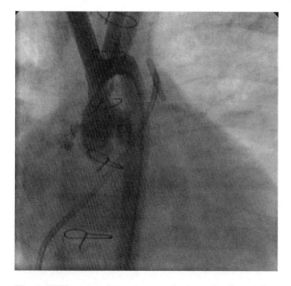

Fig. 1 Williams syndrome supravalvar aortic obstruction

procedure, but should be considered when RV pressure is above systemic and the patient has multiple stenoses proximally and distally.

A catheter is then advanced to the distal pulmonary artery. This may require the use of the bent end of a stiff wire with an appropriate "PA curve" advanced to the end of (but not out of) the catheter. Otherwise, a torque wire, or a Cook wire may be used. The branch pulmonary artery with less significant stenosis is usually entered first. A wedge pressure and free PA pressure are recorded, with attention to the mean PA pressure. If lobar obstructions are suspected, a hand injection in the free position may be recorded to show the location of pressure measurement. The pullback is then continued to the MPA. At this point remember to note if there is a diastolic gradient from the MPA to RV indicating pulmonary valve function.

The catheter is then advanced to the contralateral, more obstructed PA. A position in the lower lobe of that lung is desirable. A saturation and pressure measurement in that location is done, possibly followed by a hand injection to show location. Next, a 0.035″ Rosen wire (or other exchange length wire) is advanced as distally as possible into the lower lobe. The end-hole catheter is withdrawn. Angiography follows.

Baseline Angiography

This can be done by changing your short sheath for a long sheath and doing injections through that. Alternatively, a pigtail catheter may be advanced over the wire to the PA in the area of suspected obstruction and a Y-adapter used. In smaller patients the combination of an 0.018″ torque wire or an 0.025″ exchange Amplatz wire with a 5 F cut pigtail catheter works. A Y-adapter is then attached over the wire to the pigtail catheter and the other port is attached to the transducer. At this point you can also perform a pullback pressure assessment over the wire. To do this the hemostat valve of the Y-adapter over the wire is loosened just enough to allow easy pullback of the catheter over the wire (without altering the pressure waveform). While maintaining wire tip position in the distal

PA a pullback pressure recording is done from the distal PA to the MPA, RV, and RA. The catheter is then re-advanced over the wire into the distal PA. Recognize that the holes of the pigtail are distributed over a fair distance, so you will not be able to precisely localize the obstruction unless you use an end-hole catheter.

The port of the Y-adapter is then attached to the injector. It is important that the hemostat over the wire be tightened to prevent recoiling of the catheter or injection of the wire into the heart during injection. The wire should also be held during injections. Obtain an angiogram of the pulmonary artery with the catheter positioned so that contrast is injected just proximal to the area of stenosis. In the presence of severe pulmonary regurgitation, the catheter can be positioned more distally allowing regurgitation of contrast to show the proximal anatomy. The first angiogram is usually done in the straight PA and lateral projections Fig. 2. If needed, the cameras can then be repositioned to optimally profile the area of stenosis and the angiogram repeated.

In addition to angiography to delineate the pulmonary artery anatomy, two angiograms should be considered.

1. Aortogram in the aortic arch to look for aorto-pulmonary collaterals, especially if there is additional evidence of APCs (a step-up in the oxygen saturation in the PA or

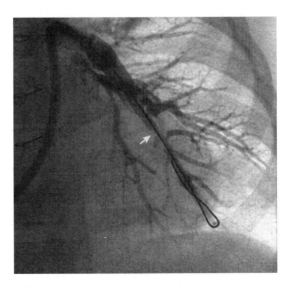

Fig. 2 Pulmonary arteries with multiple obstructions

negative wash-in on the pulmonary arterio-
gram). Stay on cine long enough to visualize
the amount of pulmonary venous return in
levophase
2. LV angiogram in patients with post-op TOF
repair to look for residual VSDs. Note that if
the RV pressure is close to systemic the angiographic diagnosis of residual VSDs can be
difficult.

Angioplasty

Based on the angiograms, the areas of stenosis
are defined in terms of location, discreteness,
and narrowest diameter. The measurements are
made by calibrating with the largest catheter in
closest proximity to the stenosis. Sometimes it
may be appropriate to calibrate using the balloon length markers.

If multiple vessels are obstructed, the largest
vessels, the most obstructed, and/or those supply-
ing the most amount of distal lung vasculature
should be considered first for dilation. Generally,
distal vessels are dilated before proximal ones,
unless the patient is particularly unstable due to
suprasystemic PA pressures.

When a vessel is chosen, wire position will be
secured across the stenosis. If the stenosis is in a
branch not along the course of the wire, then a
shaped catheter such as a or stiffer coronary
catheter sometimes cut at an angle can be used
to guide you to the pulmonary artery branch.
When you have secured wire position in the
vessel, then a balloon can be delivered to the
site of obstruction.

The choice of balloon type and size will be a
discussion for you and the primary operating physician. The appropriate size wire corresponding
to the requirements of the balloon should be positioned as distally as possible in that branch. Stiffer
wires are preferred for better tracking of the
balloon catheter. A freeze frame from the previous
angiogram is chosen that best defines the area of
stenosis and is referenced as a road map.

The balloon catheter is prepared and advanced
over the wire to straddle the area of stenosis. The
wire must be held taut with special attention paid to
its tip, so as to let go immediately if the tip starts to
be pulled back. Care is given not to allow the catheter to partially loop in the right atrium because this
tends to pull the whole apparatus backward. If this
occurs, it is resolved by quickly pulling back to
straighten the catheter or rapidly advancing the
catheter to form a complete loop in the right atrium.
If a long sheath has been placed in the PA, balloon
catheters can be passed more efficiently through the
heart. A delicate balance of advancing catheter/
pulling wire taut is needed to deliver and maneuver
the catheter to and across the area of stenosis.

When the balloon catheter is in a good position, the balloon is hand-inflated until a well-
centered waist appears. On cine the balloon is
then fully inflated by hand or with a gauge until
maximum allowable pressure or the disappearance of a waist, whichever comes first. Inflation
time is 10–60 seconds, depending on the response
of the waist, and the degree to which reduced
pulmonary blood flow and decreased cardiac output is tolerated by the patient.

You should take care not to re-cross a freshly
dilated area because of the risk of vascular injury.
The need to re-cross a freshly dilated site is
obviated by the maintenance of good distal wire
position and meticulous catheter exchanges. If re-
crossing is absolutely necessary, then a torque
wire with a soft tip is used to do this.

As already mentioned, careful inspection of
waist formation in a balloon is made during
inflation Fig. 3. No waist formation is indicative
of a very compliant vessel or an inadequately
sized balloon. If the former is true and the vessel
is quite compliant, but the diameter is
unchanged after angioplasty, then the vessel is
exhibiting recoil characteristics and may require
a stent. Recoil is much more common in proximal pulmonary arteries.

On the other extreme, a very tight waist may
herald caution that the initial choice in balloon is
too large or the vessel is resistant to conventional
balloon techniques. Note that a dilation procedure will not be successful unless the waist is
eliminated in an appropriately sized balloon. If
the waist disappears, the balloon catheter is
replaced over the wire with the cut pigtail catheter and a pullback pressure measurement and/or
angiography is done to assess the result.

If the waist does not change with a conventional angioplasty balloon, Cutting Balloon
therapy may be considered Fig. 4. A Cutting
Balloon, usually 0.5–1.0 mm larger than the

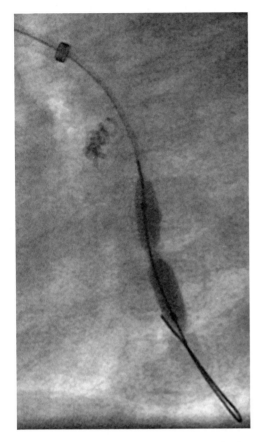

Fig. 3 Waist in balloon during pulmonary angioplasty

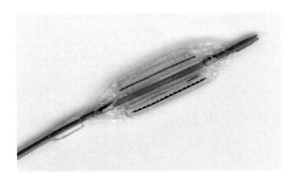

Fig. 4 Cutting Balloon

waist in the balloon and not exceeding 1 mm more than the distal PA diameter, is centered on the stenotic site. In nearly all cases, the waist will be eliminated with a Cutting Balloon. After Cutting Balloon dilation a conventional balloon the same size or slightly larger than the first balloon is used to re-dilate the site.

Angiography should be obtained between balloon inflations to screen for vessel damage.

NOTE: Pay attention, a 7 Fr sheath is required, avoid re-sheathing the balloons at an angle, and do not pull the balloon into the sheath if resistance is encountered.

An alternative in vessels that have failed "conventional" balloon dilation and that may be too large for the currently available Cutting Balloon inventory are ultra high-pressure balloons. Some of the Bard Kevlar® balloons can achieve inflation pressures up to 30 ATM. Again, balloon type and size will be determined by the operating physician.

Postcatheterization Care

Routine postcatheterization care is necessary with discharge usually planned on the next day. A chest X-ray may be helpful in assessing for postangioplasty pulmonary edema if suspected. This is most common when there is a marked increase in flow to a region that was previously protected by a tight proximal stenosis. A lung perfusion scan can quantitate the redistribution of blood flow.

Complications and Results

A procedure requiring multiple PA angioplasty is described to be among the most hazardous interventional procedures in pediatric cardiology with a mortality rate of 1% (1). However, in recent eras mortality is highly unusual. Complications of angioplasty include:

Vessel Perforation or Rupture

This results from a transmural tear, either from overdilation, catheter manipulations across a freshly dilated site, or distal catheter or wire perforation. It may manifest as acute onset of hypotension, hemoptysis, or extravasation of contrast into the pleural space or bronchi. It is managed by volume resuscitation and an attempt at balloon occlusion of the bleeding vessel proximally. The bleeding will be self-limited in some cases and require coil occlusion in others. In recent eras, we have been able to successfully manage most distal perforations successfully with coils (1).

Aneurysms

These are defined as saccular formations that taper abruptly and measure at least twice the diameter of the adjacent pulmonary artery lumen. These result from a more extensive tear in the vessel wall. In most cases this happens when the distal portion of a balloon is inflated in a very small vessel. Management is usually conservative; however, the long-term follow up of aneurysms is unknown.

Transient Pulmonary Edema

This appears to result from an acute increase in capillary perfusion pressure distal to a successfully dilated stenosis. Some patients may have hemoptysis or acute hypoxia while others remain asymptomatic. Treatment is usually conservative, i.e., oxygen and diuretics if needed, with complete resolution expected in 72 hr (2).

Results

Historically we have defined successful outcomes by one of the following criteria:

1. Greater than 50% increase in narrowest diameter.
2. More than a 20% decrease in RV/AODT pressure ratio.
3. More than a 20% increase in blood flow to the affected lung as measured by postcatheterization lung perfusion scan.

Success is expected in 50–60% of procedures using low-pressure angioplasty (3). An additional

20–30% of vessels may respond to high-pressure angioplasty if resistant to low pressures or stent therapy for compliant recoil characteristics (4,5). The remaining resistant stenosis may respond to cutting balloon therapy (6–8).

References

1. Baker C, McGowan F, Keane J et al. Pulmonary artery trauma due to balloon dilation: recognition, avoidance, and management. *J Am Coll Cardiol* 2000;36:1684–1690.
2. Arnold L, Keane J, Kan J et al. Transient unilateral pulmonary edema after successful balloon dilation of peripheral pulmonary artery stenosis. *Am J Cardiol* 1988;62:327–330.
3. Rothman A, Perry S, Keane J et al. Early results and follow-up of balloon angioplasty for branch pulmonary artery stenosis. *J Am Coll Cardiol* 1990;15:1109–1117.
4. Gentles T, Lock J, Perry S. High-pressure balloon angioplasty for branch pulmonary artery stenosis: early experience. *J Am Coll Cardiol* 1993;22:867–872.
5. Bergersen, L, Gauvreau K, Lock J et al. Recent results of pulmonary arterial angioplasty: the differences between proximal and distal lesions. *Cardiol Young* 2005;15:597–604.
6. Bergersen L, Perry S, Lock J. Effect of cutting balloon angioplasty on resistant pulmonary artery stenosis. *Am J Cardiol* 2003;91:185–189.
7. Sugiyama H, Veldtman G, Norgard G et al. Bladed balloon angioplasty for peripheral pulmonary artery stenosis. *Cathet Cardiovasc Interv* 2004;62:71–77.
8. Bergersen L, Jenkins K, Gauvreau K et al. Follow-up results of Cutting Balloon angioplasty used to relieve stenoses in small pulmonary arteries. *Cardiol Young* 2005;15:605–610.

Review Article

Bergersen L, Lock J. What is the current option of first choice for the treatment of pulmonary arterial stenosis? *Cardiol Young* 2006;16:329–338.

Balloon Dilation and Stent Placement for Coarctation

Introduction

Since its initial description in the early 1980s, balloon dilation (with or without stenting) as a treatment for coarctation of the aorta has become increasingly common, particularly outside of the neonatal period. Catheter intervention is generally recognized as the preferred method of treating recurrent coarctation. For native coarcation most centers will consider treatment of the older child or adult with primary catheter therapy, whereas balloon dilation of native coarctation in infancy is rare. Obviously, there are many diverse situations in which arch obstruction can occur, ranging from isolated coarctation with an otherwise normal heart to complex postsurgical arch obstruction following single ventricle palliation. The approach to each patient will be individualized, but there are common elements to these cases which are outlined below.

Indications for Stent Placement

Stent placement for relief of coarctation was described in the early 1990s and is now quite common across a broad spectrum of patients. At Children's Hospital Boston, predilation is performed in nearly all cases of stent placement. Patients who have failed standard balloon angioplasty or have lesions that are unlikely to resolve with balloon angioplasty alone are candidates for stent placement. Additional, rarer indications for stent placement include patients who have undergone balloon angioplasty but are left with a significant intimal tear at risk for obstruction or dissection and patients who are poor surgical candidates, either due to multiple prior operations, recent surgery, poor collateralization, or other medical conditions.

Precatheterization Considerations and Case Planning

The workup for these patients will differ somewhat depending on the type of coarctation and associated cardiac anatomy. Precatheterization information should be reviewed carefully in an effort to anticipate the aortic anatomy, degree, and nature of obstruction. Specific points to know include;

- Blood pressure, with attention to systolic hypertension and four-extremity discrepancy.
- Four extremity blood pressures should be interpreted based on arch branching, anatomy and prior catheterizations that may have resulted in femoral/iliac artery obstruction.
- Pulses, with attention to diminished femoral pulses or brachial femoral delay.
- Murmurs, which can be continuous and audible in the back.
- EKG, with attention to evidence of LVH.
- CXR looking for prominent aortic knob of evidence of rib notching.
- Doppler estimate of gradient and abdominal aortic Doppler pattern.
- Echocardiogram for LVH or increased LV mass/volume ratio.
- MRI findings if available with attention to dimensions of arch at specific points (distal, transverse, and isthmus).
- Exercise test and degree of exercise-related hypertension.

L. Bergersen et al. (eds.), *Congenital Heart Disease*,
DOI 10.1007/978-0-387-77292-9_13, © Springer Science+Business Media, LLC 2009

In patients with re-coarctation following surgery be sure to know the type of repair and if any prosthetic material was used. Anesthesia should be considered. Dilation of the aorta will be felt by the patient, and patient movement during aortic stent placement is undesirable. Discuss with your staff. A postcatheterization ICU bed is seldom needed in isolated coarctation.

Procedure and Techniques

The necessary access depends on the method chosen to measure the gradient and perform the intervention. The venous sheath should be size-appropriate for a standard right heart catheterization. If the procedure is being performed in a patient with single-ventricle anatomy, a venous sheath may be all that is necessary, although arterial monitoring in this situation is highly recommended and allows simultaneous pressure assessment above and below the area of obstruction (gold standard).

In a patient with a structurally normal heart, if you wish to record simultaneous arterial pressure tracings above and below the obstruction you'll need either two pigtail catheters (and therefore two arterial sheaths) or special catheters with two pressure transducer lumens (seldom available these days). In adult-sized patients, a second arterial sheath (4–5 Fr) may be placed in an upper extremity, which provides for simultaneous pressure recording and, more importantly, a means for good angiography during stent placement. Other techniques used to measure the gradient require only a single arterial catheter. Perhaps the most common of these involves using a sheath size 1 Fr greater than the pigtail catheter. When the standing wave is known you can obtain simultaneous measurements. Regardless of the technique used, the arterial catheter(s) should be large enough to measure an accurate pressure without excessive "fling" and to take a good aortogram.

Baseline Hemodynamics

A standard hemodynamic evaluation should be performed, focusing not only on the arch gradient but also upon cardiac sequelae of arch obstruction (mixed venous saturation, ventricular end-diastolic pressure, etc.). The coarctation gradient can be grossly estimated with the standard pigtail pullback. Following this, a precise measurement of the coarctation gradient is desirable by one of the methods described above. This is fairly straightforward in single-ventricle patients (before Fontan) by simultaneous retrograde and antegrade approaches. Otherwise, if you are using the pigtail/short sheath mismatch method you will need to account for any pulse wave amplification ("standing wave") because the femoral arterial systolic pressure is normally higher than that obtained in the thoracic aorta. To do this place a pigtail catheter through a short sheath that is 1–2 Fr sizes larger. Record a pressure with the catheter just beyond the tip of the sheath in the iliac artery, with superimposed tracings confirming well-balanced transducers. Next, advance the pigtail to just below the obstruction and re-measure. There should be a difference. This is your standing wave, calculated as follows:

*eqalign*Standing wave = femoral artery systolic pr
$$- \text{dAo systolic pressure}$$

Now, advance the catheter to just above the obstruction. Record your gradient and calculate the arch gradient as follows:

Arch gradient = (aAo systolic pressure
$$- \text{femoral artery systolic pressure})$$
$$+ \text{standing wave}$$

If you do not account for the standing wave, a simultaneous AoAs and iliac artery trace will underestimate the gradient.

When the gradient is determined, angiography is performed, usually through a pigtail catheter. Camera positions should be straight AP (sometimes with caudal) and lateral. If the coarctation is very tortuous and poorly visualized on the initial cine, the cameras can be adjusted accordingly prior to repeating angiography. Measure the narrowest part of the lesion as well as the size of the lumen immediately proximal and distal to the obstruction, and at the level of the diaphragm. Make note of relative positions of brachiocephalic vessels and any visible collaterals.

At this point the pigtail catheter is removed and suitable wire position is established. We

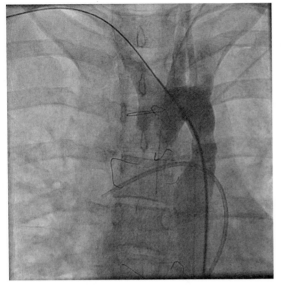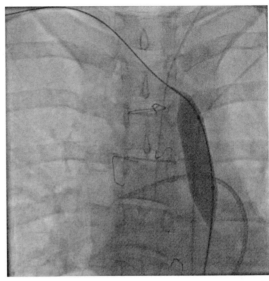

Fig. 1 Balloon dilation of coarctation

prefer relatively stiff exchange-length wires (e.g., Amplatz Super Stiff) whose tip can be either in the subclavian artery, the ascending aorta, or, rarely, the LV. With distal wire position in the LV, ectopy may be an issue, and with position in the AoAs care must be taken to keep free of the coronary ostia. Either subclavian artery provides a "worry-free" position for the distal wire, although the caliber of the left subclavian needs to be large enough to house the inflated balloon, if the wire goes into this vessel. Thus, given these considerations we almost always position the wire in the right subclavian artery.

When considering the length of the balloon it is important to have good stability, but the balloon should not be so long or of such a long taper that full inflation is impeded by the natural curvature of the aortic arch. Initial dilation, whether antegrade or retrograde, is performed with relatively dilute contrast/saline ratios, to allow rapid balloon deflation, but be sure that you can visualize balloon waist formation and resolution Fig. 1. Following dilation, angiography is performed to assess response, tears, and other damage that may have occurred. If imaging is suboptimal in any way, adjust your views and re-image.

Choosing a Balloon

Even in cases where it seems likely a stent will be necessary, there are reasons to predilate the lesion before putting in the stent. The balloon will help to verify your lesion measurements and assess the stability of balloon positioning during inflation and the compliance of the lesion. Balloon size is based on the measured diameter of the lesion and will be discussed by you and your attending. A standard first balloon is two to three times the minimal diameter of the lesion without exceeding ~1.2 times the diameter of the surrounding aorta.

Stenting

The balloon diameter for stenting is usually 1–2 mm larger than was used for predilation if the predilation balloon permitted full inflation. Obviously, if a stent is to be mounted on the balloon, the balloon needs to be longer than the stent. A smaller stent length/balloon length ratio allows more insurance against stent migration either in transit to the lesion or during balloon inflation, but significant balloon overlap in larger balloons can cause a significant "dumb-bell" deformity of the stent during inflation. Most commonly we use a relatively noncompliant balloon for dilation and stent placement (see the Appendix). Balloon-in-balloon (BIB) catheters can also be used to place the stent (by reassessing position after full inflation of the inner balloon) and may prevent excessive "dog-boning" of the stent.

In order to deliver the stent to the coarctation, we always exchange for a long sheath. The size of the long sheath is determined by the size of the balloon/stent combination. When the sheath is in place and the dilator has been removed, the stent should be readied (see section on loading stents). The most important part of stent selection is to ensure that it can be ultimately dilated up to an adult size (i.e., at least 18 mm), or else you may be committing the patient to future surgical intervention on the arch. This may be unavoidable, but it should always be considered and the options discussed with the medical and surgical teams involved.

The length of stent chosen will be based on the length of coverage needed within the lesion. Some stents will shorten significantly when expanded. Charts are available which give typical lengths for each type of stent over a range of expanded diameters (see the Appendix). The stent should be placed coaxially on the balloon and firmly apposed to the balloon without overlap of any struts. Generally, the stent is loaded in the center of the balloon, between the radiopaque shaft markers.

A well-crimped stent will not migrate forward or backward along the length of the balloon despite being introduced through the sheath, manipulated within the body, or gently pulled and pushed with your fingertips. Actual placement of the stent will be guided by previous angiographic images as well as several small hand injections of contrast through the long sheath, in an attempt to avoid unnecessary overlapping/jailing of branch vessels. In cases of significant poststenotic dilation it may be difficult to get a good angiogram through the sheath after the stent has been partially uncovered. Allowing for a little extra room in the sheath will aid angiography. The balloon is then inflated, typically by hand, deploying the stent, and then rapidly deflated Fig. 2.

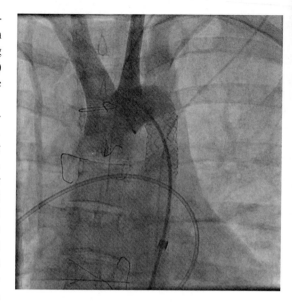

Fig. 2 Stent placement in coarctation

Finishing Up

After stenting, the gradient is measured and another angiogram is taken. Pay particular attention to sites where there may be subintimal or extravascular contrast. If there is any doubt, then another angiogram from a different angle should be obtained. Angiograms may be performed via a pigtail catheter or through the long sheath. Meticulous attention should be paid to the ACT and the long sheath. Long sheaths easily form a nice stagnant column of blood that will quickly clot. Injections performed through the sheath, if there is a clot, will have undesirable results. Do **not** let this happen!

Postcatheterization Care

These patients are admitted overnight. They receive one dose of antibiotic at the time of stent placement and during hospitalization. Most operators do not treat with heparin, but aspirin is frequently recommended for 6 months. When the patient is mobile, a PA and lateral chest film documents the placement of the stent prior to discharge. Be sure to obtain a new set of four-extremity blood pressures.

Results and Complications

Balloon dilation of coarctation in children during the first several months of life remains controversial, because while often acutely successful, restenosis is common (60–80%) and femoral artery trauma remains a significant issue. Re-stenosis rates decrease over the first year of life and this procedure is still occasionally performed in critically ill neonates. Stenting is typically avoided in young children.

At Children's Hospital Boston (1,2) the acute results of aortic stenting are good in patients aged 6 days to 60 years (mean 15.8 years), with a residual gradient greater than or equal to 20 mmHg in less than 5% of patients. In our first 153 patients, the peak to peak gradient was reduced from 30 mmHg to 0 mmHg (not including patients with systemic arteriopathy). Lumenal diameters increased by almost 50%.

Operators may intentionally stage the procedure in severe obstructions; partially dilating the coarctation region/stent then fully expanding the stent 6 months to a year later. Re-intervention, primarily redilation of the stent, is relatively common. Freedom from re-interventon is 50% at 5 years in our experience. Need for reinterrention is due to a combination of factors, including:

1. redilation to account for somatic growth in young/small patients;
2. "staged" therapy for patients with severe obstruction, whereby the stent is not expanded aggressively at the time of placement; and
3. recurrent/residual obstruction.

Our experience has suggested that elevated end-diastolic pressures, frequently associated with even mild coarctation, are reduced following effective stenting. Redilation of stents with successful expansion may be performed, even 5 or more years after placement.

Neurologic injury and uncontrolled aortic tear/rupture are uncommon but potentially devastating complications of coarctation stenting. Aortic aneurysms and dissections are also potential complications of coarctation dilation/stenting, although together they have been observed acutely in only 2% of our patients, and at the time of follow-up catheterization in 6% of patients. The long-term significance of such injuries is unknown, but we are not aware of progression to rupture in our patient population.

References

1. Marshall AC Perry SB, Keane JF et al. Early results and medium term follow-up of stent implantation for mild residual or recurrent aortic coarctation. *Am Heart J* 2000; 139:1054–1060.
2. Qureshi AM, McElhinney DB, Lock JE et al. Fifteen years of stent implantation for coarctation of the aorta: acute and intermediate outcomes and evaluation of aortic wall injury. *Cardiol Young* 2007; 17: 307–318.

RV-PA Conduit Dilation and Stenting

Introduction

A number of congenital heart lesions, most frequently those in association with pulmonary atresia, are surgically corrected with the use of right ventricle-to-pulmonary artery (RV-PA) conduits. Conduits may be synthetic, or more commonly valved pulmonary, aortic homografts, or bovine jugular grafts. Over time the conduits become calcified, the valves become dysfunctional, and there is resulting stenosis and/or regurgitation. While many centers address conduit stenosis through surgical replacement, transcatheter conduit dilation and/or stenting can delay the need for surgery by several years (1,2). While it is tempting to view the physiology of right ventricular outflow tract obstruction in this situation as analogous to simple valvar pulmonary stenosis (indeed the obstruction is often at the conduit valve), the underlying anatomy and pathophysiology are substantially different and the technical aspects bear little resemblance.

Precatheterization Considerations and Case Planning

- Pay attention to the history of previous surgical procedures and catheterization interventions including the size and type of conduit and any conduit augmentation, coronary anatomy, and prior proximal PA interventions.
- Among other findings, the CXR will reveal the degree of conduit calcification.
- An echocardiogram should estimate RV pressure and function, site, and severity of conduit obstruction, and residual cardiac defects if present. Presence of an atrial or ventricular level defect is important as is the degree of TR. A Doppler of the TR jet is the best estimation of RV pressure and therefore the degree of conduit obstruction.
- A lung scan will help to determine distribution of pulmonary blood flow.
- In some cases, a cardiac MRI adds information about anatomy, RV function, quantitative pulmonary regurgitant fraction, and RV volume.

Dilation and stenting of isolated conduit obstruction does not usually require anesthesia or a postcatheterization ICU bed. Exceptions are likely in situations of very elevated RVp or ventricular dysfunction.

Procedure and Techniques

Hemodynamics

Initial hemodynamics can be obtained through a standard short venous sheath. An arterial sheath is chosen of appropriate size to permit good quality aortic or selective coronary angiograms if necessary. Standard right and usually left heart hemodynamics is performed. A precise and accurate measurement of the RV-to-Ao pressure ratio is imperative. Balancing the transducers with the catheters in these positions verifies the accuracy of the ratio.

NOTE: Early warning signs of a sick patient are low SVC saturations, unexpectedly high mean RAp, prominent RA *a* waves (suggestive of severe RV hypetrophy and hypertension), or prominent RA *v* waves (suggestive of hemodynamically important TR).

L. Bergersen et al. (eds.), *Congenital Heart Disease*,
DOI 10.1007/978-0-387-77292-9_14, © Springer Science+Business Media, LLC 2009

Caution: *In rare cases of severe suprasystemic RV pressure and/or severe RV dysfunction, one should consider probing for an atrial septal defect, because an atrial defect can support cardiac output during complete RVOT obstruction during dilations.*

A catheter is advanced from the RV to the MPA. **Note:** This can be quite challenging in some patients, due to the often very muscular trabeculated RV, the orientation of the conduit, and the presence of free PR. In some patients, the usual advance with clockwise rotation from the RV outflow will successfully find the conduit. In others, a right atrial loop, a shaped stiff wire with an "S" bend, or a shaped catheter is necessary. Probing randomly with a torque wire out the tip of a wedge catheter in the RV is likely to result in ectopy and is unlikely to find any useful position into the PAs.

A brief stop in the MPA (with the balloon taken down) can give you a quick conduit gradient without worrying about the contribution of gradients into either PA. Also pay attention to the diastolic gradient from the RV to MPA (full ventricularization of the MPA diastolic trace may be seen in "free" PR). Alternatively, or if you skip this, the catheter is advanced into the left or right PA. A routine simultaneous systemic ventricular pressure and wedge pressure are obtained with pullback gradients to the proximal branch PA and MPA. Measurements are then repeated on the other side. Note any gradients to either PA that may need further characterization. Finally, do your pullback from the left ventricle to the aAo and dAo to get your catheter away from the carotid arteries.

At this point you will probably want to better characterize where along the conduit (or above it, or below it) your gradient is distributed. This can be done a number of ways ranging from a simple direct pullback with the end-hole, or by pulling a multipurpose catheter or long sheath over a wire. Either way, stop at areas of pressure change and do a quick hand injection to document the location.

Angiography

When you have completed your hemodynamic assessment you are ready to take your angiograms, including RV or conduit (as appropriate) and any other angiograms as needed. For example, Consider LV for residual VSD if LVp > RVp, branch PAs, if obstruction is suspected by pressure measurement, and selective coronary angiography if there is a risk that you may compress a coronary with a conduit stent. The RV-PA conduit is usually best seen in the lateral projection, but also may be visualized well in a PA with cranial angulation.

Based on the angiograms, the areas of stenosis are defined in terms of location, length, and narrowest diameter. The measurements are made via auto-calibration or by calibrating with the largest catheter in closest proximity to the stenosis. Place an end-hole or other catheter in a lower lobe PA and position an appropriately shaped exchange-length wire (usually a Rosen or Super Stiff). Remove the catheter over the wire, leaving it in position.

Balloon Dilation and Stenting

With very rare exceptions conduit dilation should occur prior to stenting, and therefore at this point a balloon is chosen and your sheath is changed for either a short sheath of appropriate size or a long sheath that allows for quick angiography (and stent placement) Fig 1. We usually choose balloons based on the initial size and

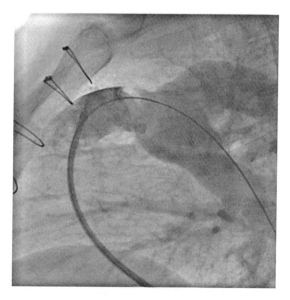

Fig.1 Angiogram of RV to PA conduit

current appearance of the conduit, with a balloon diameter up to but not exceeding 110% of the nominal conduit diameter. A noncompliant balloon, capable of inflation at high pressure, is usually selected. The balloon is prepared with dilute contrast in order to allow visualization but also rapid deflation. The balloon is advanced over the wire to straddle the area of stenosis.

When the balloon catheter is in a good position, the balloon is hand inflated until a well-centered waist appears. On cine the balloon is then fully inflated by hand or with a gauge until maximum allowable pressure, or the disappearance of a waist, whichever comes first. Careful inspection of waist formation in the balloon is made during inflation. A very tight waist may herald caution that the initial choice in balloon is too large. Also pay close attention to the ends of the balloon as the balloon straightens out.

Often, conduits are heavily calcified and in the shape of an arch as they course over the heart to the branch PAs. As such, as the balloon straightens with inflation it can have significant effects remote from your intended waist. Quickly take the balloon down (deflate) and advance it (quickly but carefully) into a branch PA or back into the RV or RA to allow the patient to recover. Try to fully deflate the balloon before drawing it back through the tricuspid valve. Remove the catheter over the wire, leaving the wire in position. Advance a cut-off pigtail over the wire with a Y-adapter on the end or use the long sheath to perform the necessary angiography. Look for improved diameter, any concerning extravascular contrast, and then check your gradient again.

Often, balloon dilation of the conduit is insufficient to relieve the obstruction and stenting is required. Accordingly, an appropriately sized stent is chosen with your attending, taking into account that most larger stents shorten from their original length based on the diameter of the balloon used to dilate.

There are two different ways to deliver the stent (see the section on "How to Load a Stent") one of which will be chosen based on your individual circumstances and attending preference. With either method, a long sheath is used to cover the stent/balloon combination as the position is obtained. If there is any residual valve function, try to avoid stenting over the valve,

although this is often not possible because the obstruction is usually at the level of the valve. With the stent in precise position the sheath is retracted, uncovering the stent and balloon.

Hand injections can be performed through the side arm of the sheath to confirm position. When you are sure that you are where you want to be, the balloon is inflated and the stent is thereby deployed Fig 2. The balloon is quickly deflated and repositioned to permit the patient's recovery. *Be careful* moving the sheath through the newly deployed stent as you recapture the balloon, particularly if you think that it is not yet entirely secure. You do not want to dislodge it! At this point, repeat angiography is performed and further dilation (or stent placement) can occur Fig 2. A final pressure measurement is made and you should be done.

Postcatheterization Care

Antibiotics are routinely administered in addition to routine postcatheterization care, a chest X-ray should be performed on the night of the catheterization to confirm stent position, exclude increased heart size or pleural effusions, and provide a new "baseline" film. A lung perfusion scan can be done if you dilated proximal or branch PAs.

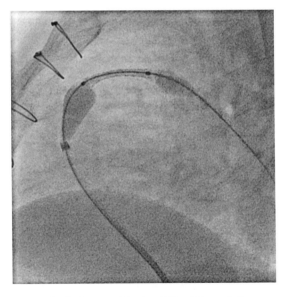

Fig. 2 Stent positioning RV to PA conduit

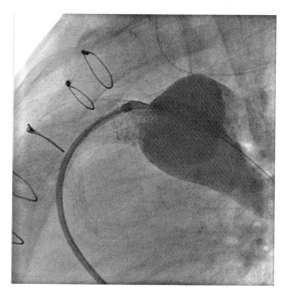

Fig. 3 Angiogram after stent placement

Results and Complications

In 15 years of experience with this procedure more than 220 patients have had conduit stents placed at Children's Hospital Boston (1,2). On average there is a 32% reduction in RV-PA pressure gradients, with RV/Ao pressure ratios dropping from 91% to 58%. Freedom from conduit surgery is 2.7 (*median*) years overall and almost 4 years in patients >5 years old.

There have been no deaths, strokes, or myocardial infarctions. Contained contrast extravasation does occasionally occur. Only one patient had a late-recognized (in recovery) conduit rupture requiring ECMO and urgent surgery. Stent malposition and embolization occurred rarely (~4%) and were more common in our early experience. Half of these were managed in the catheterization lab without a need for surgery. Predilation of the conduit before stent placement is important in minimizing stent malposition. Excluding the potential for coronary compression is imperative when contemplating stent therapy. Asymptomatic stent fracture has been identified on follow-up evaluation in at least 43% and appears more common when the conduit is immediately beneath the sternum (being compressed by the heart and sternum).

References

1. Powell AJ, Lock JE, Keane JF et al. Prolongation of RV-PA conduit life span by percutaneous stent implantation intermediate results. *Circulation* 1995; 92:3282–3288.
2. Peng L, McElhinney DB, Nugent AW et al. Endovascular stenting of obstructive right ventricle to pulmonary artery conduits: a 15-year experience. *Circulation* 2006;113:2598–2605.

The Pre-Glenn and Pre-Fontan Catheterization

Introduction

Single-ventricle physiology is a very general description, as there are many types of patients with single ventricles, and the physiology of these patients changes as they undergo surgical palliation (usually via Norwood/Sano, Glenn, and Fontan operations). Catheterizations frequently are performed preoperatively to ensure that the hemodynamics are suitable for surgery, to further define anatomy, and to intervene on lesions that could be problematic at the time of surgery, in the immediate postoperative period, or in the long-term.

What Makes Good Single-Ventricle Physiology

Indicators of good single-ventricle physiology include normal pulmonary artery architecture, low pulmonary areteriolar resistance, a well-functioning and unobstructed ventricle, and no shunts contributing to ineffective pulmonary blood flow, ventricular volume loading, or cyanosis. In the pre-Glenn/pre-Fontan catheterization these requirements are specifically assessed.

Low-Resistance Pulmonary Circulation

Pulmonary arteriolar resistance is extremely important in these patients and you need to be able to measure the PVR. The trans-pulmonary gradient (mean PA pressure–mean LA pressure) divided by the indexed pulmonary flow (Qp) will give you the PVR. (See the chapter on hemodynamic in Part I). Also pay close attention to any gradient, if present, across pulmonary veins or residual ASD.

Well-Functioning, Unobstructed Ventricle

The function of the ventricle is collectively determined by precatheterization echocardiography, ventricular diastolic pressure, cardiac output, and contractility by angiography. Outflow tract obstruction can be assessed by direct pressure pullback or simultaneous ventricle and aorta pressure measurements.

No Volume Overload

Problems include AVV regurgitation and systemic to pulmonary artery shunts or collaterals.

No Extracardiac Right-to-Left Shunts.

Possible shunts include systemic venous to pulmonary venous collaterals and pulmonary AVMs.

Precatheterization Considerations and Case Planning

Most of these cases are performed with conscious sedation. Access is usually via the femoral vessels with a second venous line from above (LSCV or RIJV) in pre-Fontan patients to access the pulmonary arteries. Both IJ and SCV lines can be distressing to the patient, no matter how quickly or easily access is achieved, and in a moving patient these areas may be difficult to keep sterile. Additional sedation or anesthesia may be necessary for some patients. Postcatheterization ICU beds are seldom necessary and early cases not requiring interventions may be considered for same-day discharge.

L. Bergersen et al. (eds.), *Congenital Heart Disease*,
DOI 10.1007/978-0-387-77292-9_15, © Springer Science+Business Media, LLC 2009

Procedure and Techniques

Hemodynamics

Obtain saturations for estimation of pulmonary (Qp) and systemic (Qs) flow. Recalling the important factors for good single-ventricle physiology, assess your pressure measurements critically. Remember, obstruction can occur at any level, and gradients of 1–2 mmHg can be significant in a venous pathway.

Systematically, with careful pressure recordings, rule out gradients at all levels.

1. Surgical anastomosis sites; SVC to PA post-Glenn.
2. Ventricular outflow, Stansel or arch obstruction.
3. Proximal and peripheral pulmonary arteries.
4. Pulmonary veins; measure bilateral PA wedge to ventricular diastolic/LA pressure or direct pulmonary vein to LA pressure pullback measurements.
5. Atrial septum; measure pullback from LA to RA.
6. AV valve stenosis; will cause a wedge-ventricle diastolic pressure gradient; you can also compare the atrial *a* wave or mean pressure and the ventricular end diastolic pressure.

A Few Things to Remember

- Particularly in these cases, the baseline blood gas should be reviewed prior to obtaining hemodynamic data. Oversedation and/or hypoventilation and resultant respiratory acidosis will adversely effect measurements.
- As a corollary, occluded access sites should be known, and access should be obtained quickly so as to minimize the likelihood of excessive sedation.
- When a left subclavian line is used and there are two operators at the table, having one person stand on the left of the table can expedite catheter manipulations and reduce radiation exposure to the operator on the right by not having to reach across the patient.
- In patients with a Glenn, there is no true mixed venous saturation. By convention, we use the SVC saturation as the mixed venous saturation for hemodynamic calculations.
- For patients with a BT shunt (and no other means of pulmonary blood flow) PA saturations should equal the aortic saturation. If there are dual sources of pulmonary blood flow (through a shunt or Glenn plus the native pulmonary artery or significant collaterals) you cannot estimate pulmonary blood flow by Fick (nor therefore PVR) without test occluding one source.
- In shunted single ventricles, the BTS is crossed with a cut-off pigtail catheter. You can cross a Sano RV-to-PA conduit with either a balloon end-hole or shaped catheter such as a Judkins right coronary catheter.
- If you do not wish to cross the BT shunt or Sano connection during a pre-Glenn catheterization you can estimate PA pressure from pulmonary venous wedge pressure, but note that this is only an accurate estimate if the venous wedge is <15 mmHg.
- If possible, measure your transpulmonary gradient (mean PAp to mean pulmonary vein pressure difference) simultaneously, i.e., catheters in PA and PV.

Angiography

Pulmonary Angiography

This is usually performed in straight AP and lateral projections Fig 1. The Qp/Qs and pulmonary anatomy determine the amount of contrast required. Remember to note PA size, anastomotic sites, distortion of PAs from prior band or shunt, branching pattern, wash-in (APCs), transit time to levophase (AVMs), pulmonary venous return, and clearance across the atrial septum.

Pulmonary AVMs are characterized by rapid opacification (<3 beats) of the LA on PA angiography together with a spongiform (also described as "salt-and-pepper" or stippled) appearance in the affected areas of the lung. Suspected AVMs should be further assessed by measuring pulmonary vein saturations, which are significantly decreased in affected areas of the lung and do not fully normalize on 100% FiO_2.

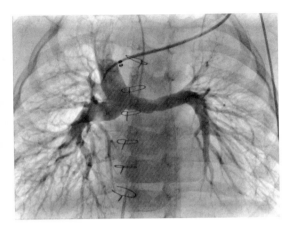

Fig. 1 Glenn pathway angiogram

regurgitation, and any evidence of dyskinesis or aneurysm. Use a pigtail retrograde from the artery or Berman antegrade. If AV valve regurgitation is being assessed the angiogram should be performed retrograde. Projection varies depending on anatomy.

Interventions

Interventions are based on the findings and the patient's clinical condition, and may include occlusion of collateral vessels or angioplasty/stents to relieve obstructions.

Aortogram

An aortogram should demonstrate any evidence of native or neoAR, coronary arteries, arch anatomy, location of shunt, and aortopulmonary collaterals if present.

Systemic Veins

The presence of an LSVC or systemic venous-to-pulmonary venous connections can be assessed with a balloon occlusion angiogram in the innominate (left usually) vein with hand injection. If the patient has significant and yet unexplained cyanosis, look for other venous collaterals from the right-sided veins (RIJV, RSCV) and even IVC and hepatics.

Ventriculogram

A ventriculogram can be performed to assess single-ventricle systolic function, AV valve

Postcatheterization Care

A hematocrit may be obtained 6 hr postcatheterization if there is a significant amount of blood loss during the case or unexplained clinical deterioration. If a BT shunt is crossed, we routinely run heparin overnight (20 U/kg/hr, max 750 U/hr) and resume aspirin as an outpatient. Other care depends on any interventions performed.

Results and Complications

The most common complication in a pre-BDG catheterization is blood loss requiring blood transfusion, so avoid unnecessary blood loss at all times. Sustained arrhythmias are not common. Beware of thrombosis after crossing BT shunts. Pneumothoraces or hemothoraxes may complicate subclavian access.

Device Closure of Fontan Fenestrations

Introduction

Since the late 1980 s, essentially all Fontan operations at Children's Hospital Boston have been done using a *fenestrated* technique. The rationale behind this modification is as follows: For a Fontan circulation to function properly, it is critical that the pulmonary vascular resistance be low and that the mean PA pressures also be low. In particular, it is desirable to have a mean PA pressure below 20 mmHg. Cardiopulmonary bypass invariably results in an increase in PVR in the immediate postoperative period. To increase cardiac output and possibly reduce the pressure in the Fontan pathway, a small hole is created in the Gore-Tex baffle that makes up part of the lateral tunnel. This fenestration is 4 mm in diameter and is directed anteriorly and leftward. It allows some of the systemic venous return to enter the systemic circulation (right-to-left shunt across the baffle) and bypass the lungs. This results in maintenance of forward cardiac output at the expense of oxygen saturation. The fenestration technique has resulted in a much more stable postoperative ICU course as well as a decreased incidence and duration of pleural effusion following Fontan surgery (1).

Patients with extracardiac Fontan procedures can also be fenestrated by the surgeon, although these fenestrations do seem to spontaneously occlude more unpredictably, often early in the postoperative course. The location of these fenestrations is more variable, often either inferiorly or superiorly as the conduit courses near the right atrial free wall, and some surgeons will interpose a small tube graft between the conduit and the lateral right atrium. The procedure described for closure is similar to that for lateral tunnels. It is also worth noting that fenestration is not universal among institutions, with much variability from center to center.

While the fenestration is certainly of benefit in the immediate postoperative period, it becomes a liability afterward. Some fenestrations will undergo spontaneous closure, but many do not. A persistent fenestration allows systemic desaturation and possible "paradoxical emboli." It has been our practice to close these fenestrations in patients with good hemodynamics a year or more after Fontan (2,3).

Precatheterization Considerations and Case Planning

Most Fontan patients presenting for fenestration closure are toddlers or preschoolers. Your precatheterization assessment should include consideration of their clinical status and the usual medical and surgical historical details. The patient's systemic saturation in clinic in conjunction with his or her echocardiogram will give you insightful information. The mean gradient across the fenestration should be approximately equal to the transpulmonary gradient. If the echocardiogram shows a "tiny" fenestration but the patient's saturations are in the 70 s, other reasons for cyanosis will need to be sought.

Procedure and Techniques

Since these patients are generally larger than 20 kg you will probably start with a 7 Fr sheath in the vein and either a 4 Fr or 5 Fr sheath or pigtail catheter in the artery. Sometimes a

L. Bergersen et al. (eds.), *Congenital Heart Disease*,
DOI 10.1007/978-0-387-77292-9_16, © Springer Science+Business Media, LLC 2009

second 4 Fr or 5 Fr venous line will be used for baffle angiography during device positioning and simultaneous pressure measurement in the fontan pathway. Access is obtained via the femoral vessels, a baseline ACT is drawn and heparin is given.

Hemodynamics

Saturations and pressures are obtained by a pull-back from the SVC to the baffle and usually to the IVC. NOTE: *special attention is paid to any venous gradients because even 1–2 mm of gradient can be significant.* The arterial catheter is advanced retrograde into the ventricle, and LPA and RPA capillary wedge pressures are simultaneously compared to the ventricular diastolic pressure tracing. A discrepancy in the wedge–diastolic pressure measurement indicates potential stenosis of the pulmonary veins, AV valve, atrial septum, or the presence of significant AP collaterals. The catheter in the ventricle is then pulled back to the level of the diaphragm, noting any gradients from the ventricle to ascending aorta or across the arch. Pullbacks are obtained from the LPA and RPA to the baffle to evaluate the proximal branch pulmonary artery connections.

The fenestration is crossed by probing the lateral wall of the baffle with a Berman catheter if a single venous line is used and a balloon end-hole catheter if two lines are present. A stiff wire with a hockey stick bend at the end may be inserted into the catheter to facilitate catheter direction toward the fenestration. Alternatively, a shaped catheter can be used and the hole can be probed with a torque wire. A baffle angiogram (PA, lateral) will identify the fenestration location (if present) and other leaks (if present). When the fenestration is identified and crossed, an LA saturation is drawn and pressure is measured. If there is evidence of LA desaturation, individual pulmonary veins should be entered and saturations measured.

Fenestration Test Occlusion

Because the Berman catheter holes are proximal to the balloon, the holes are actually in the baffle or RA portion of the Fontan pathway. This allows for monitoring of the Fontan pathway

saturation and pressure during test occlusion. The presence of a second line allows simultaneous measurements in the LA and baffle during test occlusion. With fenestration occlusion, the systemic arterial saturation should rise; the Fontan baffle pressure should remain constant or rise only minimally. The cardiac output may decrease evidenced by a slight drop in mixed venous saturation and rise in systemic saturation (widening the AVO difference) and a 1–2 mmHg increase in baffle pressures is common.

What constitutes "unacceptable" hemodynamic alteration is a complex clinical decision between you, the attending, and the patient's primary cardiologist. Before test occlusion, be sure to have a new baseline hemodynamic assessment (baffle pressures, Qs, etc.) Angiography can adversely affect your measurements; you do not want to attribute to fenestration occlusion alone what is truly the combined effects of angiography, a long case, *and* fenestration occlusion. At any rate, the occlusion is usually maintained for approximately 10 min while these parameters are monitored. If the occlusion is successful, it is released after 10 min and preparations are made for device closure.

Angiography

A baffle angiogram can be taken with a Berman or pigtail catheter. This angiogram should show the baffle, fenestration, and branch PAs clearly. If there are any angiographic stenoses, these should be addressed now, before proceeding with fenestration closure. The baffle angiogram will also allow for identification of any other Fontan pathway leaks. Consider taking this angiogram with the fenestration occluded. Baffle leaks around the suture line or via intramural atrial venous channels are fairly common and can be addressed with coils or with additional devices if they are large. If additional leaks are present or systemic vein to pulmonary vein connections exist, the saturation will not rise appropriately with test fenestration occlusion. Depending on the angle and location of the baffle, a second angiogram may need to be taken to show the fenestration *en face* and on edge in preparation for device closure Fig 1. For many of these patients, this will be their last "routine" catheterization. Angiography is performed to evaluate the entire Fontan and PA pathways, pulmonary venous return, ventricular function and outflow, systemic arterial obstruction, and APCs.

Fenestration Device Closure

Using the best baffle angiogram, the fenestration is identified and put up on the reference screens as a "road map". Using an end-hole catheter (wedge or other), with a stiff bent wire or torque wire, the fenestration is crossed and the catheter tip is positioned in the LA or pulmonary vein. Next, a stiff wire (often 0.035″ Rosen or Amplatz 0.035″ Super Stiff if needed) is secured in position for sheath delivery.

If you are using a CardioSEAL®, the device is inspected and then loaded into the "quick loader" at the end of the delivery system. Next, the short sheath is removed from the groin and the site is dilated with a 12 Fr short dilator. The flushed 10-F-long sheath and dilator are then advanced over the stiff wire from the RFV to the baffle, across the fenestration, and into the body of the LA. The device is loaded into the long sheath and advanced to the IVC-RA junction.

At this time, it is convenient to stop and withdraw the pusher catheter 5–8 cm, allowing the device a little more flexibility while still connected

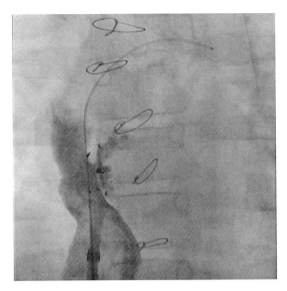

Fig. 2 Cardioseal delivered in fenestration

to the cable. The device is then advanced near the tip of the long sheath. The distal arms are delivered from the sheath in the atrium. The entire sheath/device assembly is then pulled back until the distal arms engage the LA side of the baffle and the center pin of the device is at the level of the fenestration. You must take care not to get trapped on residual atrial septum as you pull back, as this may result in incorrect deployment of the device on the wrong side of the baffle. An angiogram with the second venous line can be taken now to confirm device position. The sheath is then pulled back, allowing the proximal arms to deploy on the systemic venous side of the baffle. If the device is in good position with four arms on the atrial and four arms on the venous side of the baffle, the device is released Fig 2.

When using an AMPLATZER larger cap font as done previously in device section system, the 6- or 7-Fr-long sheath is exchanged over a wire into the LA as described above, again being careful not to entrain any air into the system. A 4-mm atrial septal occluder device is usually used, with the LA disc deployed on the systemic side of the Fontan circulation and the RA disc deployed in the Fontan baffle/conduit. Again, angiographic confirmation is used to confirm positioning and the device is released.

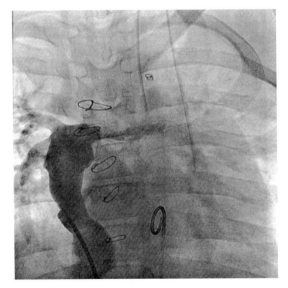

Fig. 1 Fontan angiogram showing fenestration

A final set of pressures, saturations, and baffle angiogram may be performed with attention to any gradients in relation to positioning of the device.

Postcatheterization Care

Most of these patients are admitted for observation overnight. A CXR is performed to confirm device position and provide a new baseline for future comparison. Prophylactic antibiotics are generally administered. Anticoagulation is usually recommended with either aspirin or more aggressive regimens, depending on patient risk factors.

Results and Complications

Most complications are related to the large venous access required to deliver the device. Heparin may be required postcatheterization to maintain vein patency. Device malposition or embolization is also possible, but is almost never seen in fenestration closures because the hole is only 4 mm in diameter and is in synthetic, noncontracting material. Another complication is intolerance of fenestration closure and need for subsequent refenestration. Fortunately, this too is rare.

References

1. Bridges ND. Fenestration of the Fontan baffle: Benefits and complications. *Semin Thorac Cardiovasc Surg Pediatr Card Surg Annu.* 1998;1:9–14.
2. Bridges ND, Lock JE, Mayer JE, Jr., Burnett J et al. Cardiac catheterization and test occlusion of the interatrial communication after the fenestrated Fontan operation. *J Amer Coll Cardiol.* 1995;25:1712–1717.
3. Bridges ND, Lock JE, Castaneda AR. Baffle fenestration with subsequent transcatheter closure. Modification of the Fontan operation for patients at increased risk. *Circulation.* 1990;82:1681–1689.

ASD Device Closure

Introduction

The first successful transcatheter closure of an ASD was performed by King and Mills in 1974. The device was composed of two opposing umbrellas and required a 23 Fr introducer. Since then different device designs have been studied. There are now two FDA-approved devices used for ASD closure: AMPLATZER Septal Occluder® and Helex®. Secundum atrial septal defects are usually closed to reduce right ventricular volume overload (RVVO) which is diagnosed by echo or MRI. In the presence of RVVO by noninvasive measures the ASD meets indication for closure, even when the measured Qp/Qs in the lab may suggest a less than 2:1 shunt. However, occasional patients get to the lab with a misdiagnosis or missed diagnosis, e.g., the TEE shows intact septum, multiple defects, or there are pulmonary venous anomalies, which may make ASD closure inappropriate.

Precatheterization Considerations and Case Planning

The workup for an isolated ASD is usually straightforward. Most often there is no significant past history. Ask about palpitations, any problems with coagulation (unexplained thrombosis), any contra-indication to anticoagulation (everyone will be on aspirin after the case), and allergies to antibiotics. As part of a complete physical exam, pay particular attention to S2. If there is a fixed split, this is consistent with RVVO. If it is loud, this may be evidence of raised pulmonary pressures.

You must document a good neurological exam. Check the EKG for an rSR' pattern consistent with RVVO. It is also important as a baseline, because the ASD devices can rarely cause transient or permanent conduction problems. The CXR may show increased pulmonary blood flow and a variable degree of cardiac enlargement. Look at the echocardiogram yourself. You need to know: defect size, location, rims, number of defects, and pulmonary venous anatomy. Available devices are designed to close secundum ASD and not other types of ASDs. Check for right ventricular volume overload and evidence of pulmonary hypertension. If the scheduling form does not make it clear regarding anesthesia and TEE, ask the attending. It is much better to sort out these issues the day before.

Each device has unique benefits and risks, and the type of device you will use depends in part on the size and morphology of the ASD and individual attending preference. It is sometimes helpful, and often eliminates familial confusion, if you discuss device selection with the attending before you talk to the family. If questions are asked about the available devices you should be able answer them, so some background reading is required.

Procedure and Techniques

It is *really* very difficult to deliver an ASD device from above the diaphragm (IJV or subclavian), although it can be done. If there is IVC or iliac vein occlusion or if there is an interrupted IVC, hepatic vein access may be necessary. Arterial access is nice for monitoring, but not usually necessary. If intra-cardiac echocardiography will be used, a second venous sheath can be placed.

L. Bergersen et al. (eds.), *Congenital Heart Disease*,
DOI 10.1007/978-0-387-77292-9_17, © Springer Science+Business Media, LLC 2009

Correct positioning is usually confirmed with a combination of fluoroscopy and echo. Cases using TEE are usually performed under anesthesia, which should be arranged the day before. To avoid anesthesia, intracardiac echo (ICE) also is commonly used at some centers. This requires a second 8 Fr sheath. The ICE can be performed by the catheterizer, eliminating the need for a second cardiologist (although some centers still prefer to have an echo specialist to perform the ICE). Conscious sedation is usually used for these cases. It is also possible to place the device with echo and no fluoroscopy, or with fluoroscopy and no echo!

Here is a suggested outline: Start with a femoral venous sheath large enough to accommodate the sizing balloon, a 7 Fr end-hole and a 4F 80 cm pigtail in the artery, if necessary. Give heparin and prophylactic antibiotics. Perform your hemodynamic evaluation, noting PA pressure, Qp:Qs, and atrial pressure (it should equalize if there is a decent-sized communication).

Try not to cross the ASD until the echo measurements are performed because your catheter/wire can deform the septum. When initial measurements are made you can cross the defect, pass the catheter into a left pulmonary vein, place an 0.035 Rosen wire, and slide the catheter out over the wire. An optional step before this is to perform an LA angiogram in an LAO view with cranial or caudal angulation, usually with your angiographic catheter in the RUPV. This will usually nicely detail the ASD.

Depending on the unstretched size (the stretched size is generally around 30% larger than the defect), pass a compliant 20-mm, 25-mm, or 30-mm sizing balloon over the wire. The balloon can be prepped in the IVC. Then position and inflate the balloon gently with dilute contrast while straddling the defect Fig 1. Sizing is accomplished in two ways; either "stop flow" or a circumferential waist. Know which you are using and how to apply the measurement you get to device sizing.

For the stop flow method, the inflation should be observed on the echo and stopped at the moment when the color flow around the balloon from the ASD is no longer present. For circumferential waist, be sure to achieve an indentation on both sides of the balloon in both views. If you are not careful you can pretty much make the

balloon sized measurement as big as you want, so try not to overinflate and tear the septum and make a bigger hole. While the balloon is still inflated, look at the remainder of the septum with echo for additional holes. Cine the balloon and measure the waist. Deflate the balloon and take it out. Give more lidocaine, especially if the patient is awake.

At this point you will choose your device and delivery system. Device selection is not always straightforward and involves consideration of the defect size, orientation, and other physiologic variables as well as the specific physical characteristics and performance history of the different devices. Discuss device selection with your attending.

Next, you will need to choose and prepare your long delivery sheath. It is usually a good idea not to load your device until you are ready to put the device in the body, so prepare the sheath first. Sheath size and type is another complex variable. CardioSEAL/STARflex devices usually require a significantly larger sheath then you initially used for hemodynamics, so consider predilation of the tract with a short dilator through the skin first; this makes the long sheath passage much easier.

If you are using a CardioSEAL/STARflex. a larger (14 Fr) short sheath is often placed "on the back" of the long delivery sheath. This

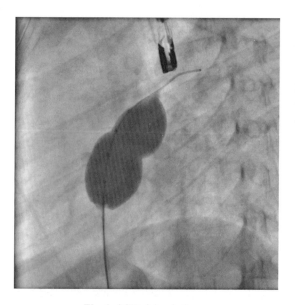

Fig. 1 ASD sizing balloon

sheath is typically left outside the body but can be inserted into the vein if necessary to remove the device. It is technically more difficult to retract a fully deployed CardioSEAL/STARflex than an AMPLATZER for reasons that become clear when you see them.

AMPLATZER delivery sheaths will range in size depending on the size of the device used. The Helex device is delivered through a 9 Fr sheath. Flush all sheaths well before placing them into the body. Now load your device into the delivery system, remove your short sheath over the wire, and carefully advance your long sheath over the wire to the LA or LPV, being extremely careful to avoid introducing air. When you are in good position, slowly remove the wire and dilator. You may prefer to leave the wire tip out the long sheath to help it from getting stuck against the roof of the LA as you withdraw the dilator. Rapid removal of either the wire or dilator will draw air into your sheath. When wire and dilator are out, make sure that the sheath is free of air either by flushing the dilator while removing under fluoroscopy or letting the sheath bleed back.

The delivery system is then advanced through the long sheath, until the device is at the end of the long sheath in the LA. In general, the device is opened by retraction of the long sheath, exposing the distal or LA component (disc or arms). When the LA component is open, withdraw everything back until the LA side is close to or just touching the septum, then retract the long sheath (leaving the center of the device in the plane of the septum) to open the RA arms/disc Fig 2. Repeat echo imaging to look at device security and its relation to the surrounding cardiac structures. If everything is correctly positioned on echo and fluoroscopy, release the device. There are fundamental differences in the deployment of different devices. For AMPLATZERs, fully appose the LA disc to the septum, to be sure that an RA disc does not open partly in the LA (the most common error). It is just the opposite for CardioSEAL/STARflex: just touch the septum with one LA arm, then open the RA arms, to avoid pulling an LA arm through (the most common error).

Prior to deployment of the RA arms of the CardioSEAL/STARFlex you can easily pull the device back into the long sheath. If the RA arms

have been opened, the device can be retrieved partially into the long sheath, but with much more difficulty and the device *will* be damaged. When the device has been brought to the IVC, it can often be partially recaptured into the long sheath. The 14 F short sheath is passed into the femoral vein, and the long sheath and device can be removed through the larger, short sheath, and access is not lost.

The AMPLATZER and Helix systems have the advantage that the whole device can be retracted easily back into the long sheath even if both discs have been opened. The device can then be repositioned and redeployed.

As suggested previously, the problematic arm with the CardioSEAL/STARFlex system is almost always the anterio-superior arm on the LA side. With the AMPLATZER, the inferior RA disc is vulnerable to malposition.

When released, the echo will document correct positioning, residual leak, and one last look for additional defects. They will also ensure that the AV valves, pulmonary veins, SVC, and IVC are not altered or obstructed. Spot cine the device *en face* and then a power injection may be performed in the RA with a 7Fr Berman or 7 Fr pigtail. Remember to stay on for levophase when the LA will also fill with contrast. Look at device position and residual leak.

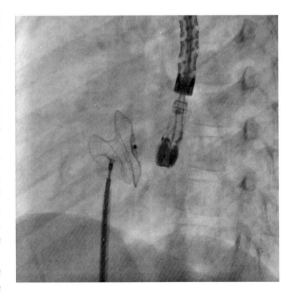

Fig. 2 AMPLATZER ASD device delivery

The lateral camera profiles the plane of the atrial septum, thus confirming correct position, while the AP camera (perpendicular) shows the size of the atrium and demonstrates the relationship to AV valves, and systemic and pulmonary veins. At the end, place the cameras in straight AP and lateral for a spot cine. This is used for comparison with the CXR taken later if there are any concerns.

Postcatheterization Care

Anticoagulation requirements after placement of the device are not well understood, and therefore there are no standards across patients or operators. However, almost all physicians will prescribe aspirin. Variations include aspirin prior to and the evening of the case, Plavix[®], overnight heparin, and sometimes coumadin. Following the proceeding we routinely check a hematocnt and CXR. Prophylactic antibiotics are generally administered. The CXR should confirm that the device is in the identical position as that documented in the lab. The next morning you can obtain an EKG and Echo prior to discharge with aspirin for 6 months (+/− other anticoagulation requested).

Results and Complications

Apart from the general risks of a hemodynamic catheterization, there are some case-specific risks. Air embolization during device deployment or manipulation may be seen and can be minimized by technical vigilance. Device embolization is uncommon but can occur with any type of implantable device. Many times, this can be dealt with in the catheterization lab, although surgical retrieval may be necessary.

There are transient EKG changes in some patients. Rarely, high-grade AV block can occur, which requires intervention, especially when large devices are placed. Infection is uncommon, but periprocedural antibiotic prophylaxis is routinely used. Device thrombus has been reported with each of the devices. The AMPLATZER device has been associated with a low but not clearly known incidence of device erosion into the aorta or other surrounding structures.

Additional Readings

Zhong-Dong Du, Hijazi ZM, Kleinman CS et al. Comparison between transcatheter and surgical closure of secundum atrial septal defect in children and adults. *J Am Coll Cardiol* 2002;39:1836–1844.

Nugent AW, Britt A, Gauvreau K et al. Device closure rates of simple atrial septal defects optimized by the STARFlex device. *J Am Coll Cardiol* 2006;48:538–544.

Jones TK, Latson LA, Zahn E et al. Results of the U.S. Multicenter pivotal study of the HELEX septal occluder for percutaneous closure of secundum atrial septal defects. *J Am Coll Cardiol* 2007;49:2215–2221.

Divekar A, Gaamangwe T, Shaikh N et al. Cardiac perforation after device closure of atrial septal defects with amplatzer septal occluder. *J Am Coll Cardiol* 2005;45:1213–1218.

PFO Device Closure

Introduction

Device closure of PFO remains a relatively controversial topic in those with otherwise normal hearts. In this patient population:

- There is compelling evidence of an *association* between PFO and cerebrovascular accidents (CVA) / transient ischemic attacks (TIA), especially in patients <55 years of age, and particularly with hypermobile septum primum ("atrial septal aneurysm"). Causative data are lacking at present.
- Randomized controlled trials (RCTs) are underway, assessing the relative risks and benefits of medical therapy versus device PFO closure in addition to antiplatelet therapy in the management of stroke associated with PFO in the young. Similar RCTs are underway, assessing the relative risks and benefits of PFO closure in refractory migraneurs with large volume shunting via PFO.
- Prior HDE (humanitarian device exemption) allowance from the FDA for PFO closure when associated with recurrent stroke despite anticoagulant therapy has been halted by the FDA, making all PFO device closure for indication of stroke risk reduction currently an **off-label** use of the device, subject to individualized review and scrutiny, with unclear risks and benefits, and unclear potential for reimbursement (current status July 2008).
- A single registry (CARS) to include persons previously eligible for HDE PFO-closure for stroke risk reduction indications has had essentially no participation, and remains realistically locally unavailable.

- The most accepted indication for PFO closure in the adult is for diastolic shunting with low filling pressures, causing measurable and life-important oxygen-unresponsive hypoxemia (a variant of the so-called "orthodeoxia–platypnea" syndrome).
- Additional associations between PFO and worsened sleep apnea, decompression disease, dementia, and arrhythmia remain less well tested.

Individual catheterization operators have varying thresholds for device-based PFO closure. Patients must be aware of the off-label indication of their device for such use. It is likely that the patient and his or her family are well educated and informed regarding device closure and associated risks and benefits of alternate medical therapies. Expect that patients will have questions and that this session may be lengthy.

Precatheterization Considerations and Case Planning

The work-up is similar to ASD, especially documenting the neurological signs, pro-thrombotic risks, and in-depth evaluation of the peripheral vasculature including the presence of pules and bruits in the neck, chest, abdomen, arms, and legs. Concomitant medical confounders (diabetes control, cigarette use, atherosclerosis, body mass abnormalities, stimulant use, rheumatologic disease, immunodeficiency, chronic liver disease, renal disease, and coagulopathy) present higher potential risks and should be assessed for and documented. Record past pertinent neurologic evaluations and review of

L. Bergersen et al. (eds.), *Congenital Heart Disease*,
DOI 10.1007/978-0-387-77292-9_18, © Springer Science+Business Media, LLC 2009

imaging confirming embolization should occur. Patients are also more likely to be on anticoagulation, so ask when the last dose was and check coagulation studies before the procedure.

Many devices have nickel within their alloy, and the occurrence of nickel allergy has been reported, albeit in rare circumstances. Allergy history should be discussed. Although also uncommon in occurrence, risk of device-associated arrhythmia, thrombosis, malfunction, erosion, inflammation, and failure to protect against stroke recurrence, should all be recognized and discussed.

Procedure and Techniques

This is similar to ASD closure, with a few differences.

Because the *defect size* is often smaller. PFO's are not really "sized". The orifice can be stretched so as to better understand the relationship between the septum primum and septum secundum, as well as the relationship to adjoining atrial surfaces. Fluoroscopy alone may be sufficient. It is not unusual for PFO closure to be done with sedation and one or two venous lines, although TEE or ICE are still utilized in some cases.

An angiogram is necessary to define the anatomy of the tunnel. A common way is to do an injection with a 7 Fr cutoff pigtail over the wire coming through the PFO. An alternative way is to place a standard 7 Fr pigtail over the wire in the LA: When the wire is removed the pigtail will loop, and when withdrawn slightly the holes will lie within the PFO tunnel and the loop will stay in the LA. This gives a nice angiogram, Fig1.

When there is a long tunnel ($\geq$ 12–20 mm), some operators may puncture the *septum primum* (Brockenbrough) just inferior to septum secundum. This is to done to avoid the device deploying improperly, due to the opening being restricted by overlapping tissue that may impede apposition or capture device arms within the tunnel. Others will obtain a stretched diameter to determine the distensibility of the thin superior aspect of the septum primum and then reimage. Yet another variation is to perform a left atrial-to-right atrial balloon pull-through using a balloon end-hole catheter (inflated with ~2 cc of dilute contrast) over a wire. The idea here is to evert, or even tear

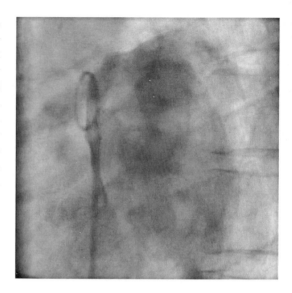

Fig. 1 PFO angiogram

portions of the septum primum, making it more incompetent, perhaps allowing improved final device position regardless of septal thickness or tunnel length. In general, most operators take both tunnel length and septal thickness into account in choosing a device size.

Postcatheterization Care

Post-device anticoagulation or antiplatelet therapy varies greatly because many of these patients will be on oral anticoagulation medicine already. In general regimens are similar to ASD's post-closure. Ask the attending what is required for each individual. Many attending physicians utilize variations of the regimens established within RCTs, i.e., preprocedural antiplatelet therapy followed by 6 months aspirin +/– 2–3 months of Plavix. Patients must be counseled prior to the procedure regarding the effects of antiplatelet therapy on bleeding or bruising, as well as the postprocedural risks of medical therapy.

Results and Complications

In a Children's Hospital Boston study using CardioSEALs in 63 patients without significant structural heart disease, 54 (86%) had effective closure of the foramen ovale (trivial or no residual shunt by echocardiography) while seven (11%) had mild and two (3%) had moderate residual shunting (1). Somewhat higher rates of closure have also been published, especially with STARFlex and BioSTAR modifications. Poor device position and the presence of an atrial septal aneurysm may increase the likelihood of residual shunt.

Reference

1. Hung J, Landzberg MJ, Jenkins KJ et al. Closure of patent foramen ovale for paradoxical emboli: intermediate-term risk of recurrent neurological events following transcatheter device placement. *J Am Coll Cardiol*. 2000;35:1311–1316.

Additional Readings

Inglessis I, Landzberg MJ. Interventional catheterization in adult congenital heart disease. *Circulation* 2007;115:1622–1633.

Mullen MJ, Hildick-Smith D, De Giovanni JV et al. BioSTAR Evaluation STudy (BEST): a prospective, multicenter, phase I clinical trial to evaluate the feasibility, efficacy, and safety of the BioSTAR bioabsorbable septal repair implant for the closure of atrial-level shunts. *Circulation*. 2006;114:1962–1967.

PDA Closure

Introduction

The first surgery for a congenital heart defect was a PDA ligation by Dr. Robert Gross (as a Chief Surgical Resident) in 1938 at Children's Hospital Boston. Since that time, therapy for PDAs has changed considerably. Catheter-directed therapy for PDA has gradually evolved since its introduction by Porstmann in 1967. In March 1992, Cambier and Moore reported an innovative adaptation in the use of Gianturco steel coils when they occluded small (<2.5 mm) PDAs in four patients. This adaptation had major advantages over previous devices in that it employed existing catheter technology, obviating the need for regulatory review and licensing. The coils were inexpensive ($20–$25 each) and could be delivered through a venous or an arterial catheter using much smaller (4 Fr) introducing sheaths. In 2003, the AMPLATZER duct occluder was the first FDA-approved device for PDA closure.

Precatheterization Considerations and Case Planning

Most of these patients have no structural heart disease so the precatheterization evaluation is usually straightforward. The exam should demonstrate the murmur of a PDA in the expected location (treatment of a "silent" PDA is controversial). The ECG and echo are usually normal (except for the PDA), but there may be evidence of for LV volume loading. Echo estimations of the PDA size should be taken as just that, estimations, but can guide case planning. Fortunately, it is unusual to see pulmonary hypertension in association with simple PDAs these days. The discussion with the family should include indications for PDA closure, which presumably eliminates / decreases the risk of infective endocarditis / endarteritis, and eliminates LV volume loading.

In planning your case consider the probable PDA size and type of closure device you will be using (coils vs. AMPLATZER ductal occluder). Equipment should include:

- A 4 Fr arterial sheath.
- Venous sheath optional (unless an AMPLATZER device is anticipated).
- A 4 Fr angiographic catheter (pigtail or Halo).
- Selection of 4 Fr end-hole catheters: Bentson / Berenstein / Cobra (all the "slimy" variety), occasionally 4 Fr multipurpose with distal holes cut off.
- Coils.
  - Coils are labeled with three numbers. For example: 38-5-4, which indicates a 0.038″ coil that is 5 cm long and that forms a 4-mm-diameter coil.
  - In general, 0.038″ coils are less floppy (but stronger with more "spring") than 0.035″ coils and are more easily seen fluoroscopically.
- Snares in the event of embolization.

Procedure and Techniques

Coil Occlusion

Strategy for closure varies from operator to operator and includes both antegrade and retrograde approaches. The retrograde approach (more stable and greater control) will be described here, as most of the technical details

L. Bergersen et al. (eds.), *Congenital Heart Disease*,
DOI 10.1007/978-0-387-77292-9_19, © Springer Science+Business Media, LLC 2009

for either approach are similar. For PDAs that are small (<2 mm) and not associated with other cardiac defects requiring hemodynamic evaluation, a single arterial catheter may be sufficient; however, a venous sheath offers an easy route to retrieve coils in the event of embolization. Right-sided hemodynamic evaluation is commonly performed from routine femoral venous access.

Femoral arterial access is obtained and a 4 Fr sheath is inserted. Heparin is administered. Hemodynamic data are recorded. An angiographic catheter is positioned in the descending aorta just distal to the expected location of the aortic ampulla of the ductus because more proximal injections tend to opacify the ascending arch of the aorta and make it more difficult to clearly see the PDA. The initial angiogram can be taken in straight PA and lateral projections. An alternative view is 35–40 degrees of RAO angulation on the PA camera. A maximum of 1 cc/kg of contrast is given rapidly; however, the small catheters used usually limit the amounts delivered.

Hand injection through the end-hole catheter can also produce a useful angiogram. The cameras should not be moved after the angiogram because the landmarks (often a tracheal air column) to be used for coil placement will depend on camera position. The narrowest portion of the PDA is then measured and compared to an *empty* catheter of known dimension (1.3 mm for a 4 Fr catheter) or the markers on a marker pigtail catheter to determine the size. The general morphology of the duct, as well as the size and length of the ampulla should also be noted. Appropriate reference images should be stored as road maps. Fig. 1.

The PDA is then crossed with a 0.035″ torque wire through one of the above end-hole catheters (usually a Berenstein with a single distal bend, a Bentson with a proximal gentle secondary curve, or a stiffer multipurpose with the tip including the side-hole cut off). With the stiff part of the torque wire straddling the ductus, the catheter is advanced over the wire into the MPA (retrograde approach). Position of the catheter in the MPA should be confirmed by pressure transduction.

A coil for occlusion is then chosen based on consideration of the duct's morphology, length, size, and patient's hemodynamics. As a general rule the coil is usually chosen to have a diameter of at least 2× the nominal diameter of the duct,

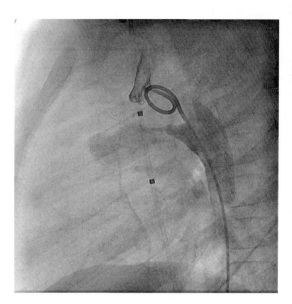

Fig. 1 PDA angiogram

and a length that will produce approximately four loops ($\pi \times$ diameter $\times$ 4) or approximately 12 × the diameter. Both 0.038″ and 0.035″ coils fit through the above catheters, and usually a 0.038″ is chosen if the appropriate size is available because it has a much stronger "spring" and is much more stable.

A straight wire (not J-tipped, not stiff) of the same caliber as the coil is advanced through the end-hole catheter into the MPA to judge the stability of the catheter position. If the catheter is stable then the coil is loaded. The metal end of the coil cartridge is placed and held firmly in the hub of the delivery catheter. The guide wire is then inserted through the plastic covered end of the cartridge, pushing the coil approximately 10–15 cm into the catheter. The empty coil cartridge is then removed over the wire and bent to designate its empty status to avoid confusion with unused cartridges.

The coil is advanced under fluoroscopy (lateral camera) to the end of the delivery catheter in the distal MPA. One-half to a single loop is extruded. The catheter and wire are then pulled back together until the loop is at the desired location at the MPA side of the ductus (use the reference image). The loop often changes orientation as it engages the ductus.

The tricky part: *The coil is now exactly where you intended; however, the aortic end is still in the*

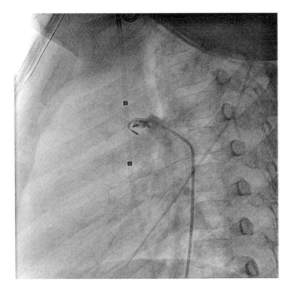

Fig. 2 PDA coil

catheter. The wire (and coil) is now kept station-ary (using the table for stabilization) as the cathe-ter is withdrawn, uncovering the aortic end of the coil Fig2. Care must be taken not to push or pull the wire / coil combination into the MPA or aorta.

The coil is now delivered, ideally with half to one loop on the MPA side, and three to three-and-a-half loops in the aortic ampulla.

A small hand injection through the end-hole catheter will indicate the magnitude of any resi-dual leak. If there appears to be a small leak at most, wait about 10 min and repeat the initial angiogram. If there is a large residual leak, con-sideration is given to re-crossing the PDA for additional coil placement.

Some other techniques include the following:

- Simultaneous delivery of 2 coils
- Bioptome-assisted delivery
- Snare-assisted delivery
- Use of 0.052″ coils

AMPLATZER *Duct Occluder*

The AMPLATZER Duct Occluder is approved for patients older than 6 months and greater than 6 kg, and is generally used only in a PDA with a minimum diameter of at least 2–2.5 mm, with a sufficiently large aortic ductal ampulla to

prevent the device from protruding out into the lumen of the descending aorta.

Venous access must be obtained for device delivery, and arterial access is used to obtain angiograms during device delivery. Initial hemo-dynamics and pictures are obtained through a short sheath. Angiography may be obtained from the venous side by passing a wire antegrade across the duct and exchanging the catheter for a pigtail catheter. Alternatively, a retrograde des-cending aortic angiogram or selective injection can be done from the arterial side.

A device is chosen in discussion with your attending, usually ~2 mm wider than the mini-mal diameter of the ductus. After a device is chosen, a long sheath ranging 6–8 French will be needed to accommodate the range of device sizes. Introduce the long sheath over a J-tipped guide wire positioned in the descending abdom-inal aorta. If an insufficient length of wire is in the Ao the stiff sheath will not make the turn through the ductus to the descending aorta.

Loading and delivering an AMPLATZER device is discussed in Part I. Be sure to have the hemostasis valve on the back of the loading catheter to prevent excessive blood loss during device delivery. The retention skirt is first deployed in the proximal descending aorta and then retracted until tension can be seen / felt against the wall of the ductus. After readvancing the pigtail, angiograms in the aorta are used to confirm device position. The device should be adjusted until it fits well in the ampulla, and then the remaining portion of the device can be deployed by unsheathing the device under tension. Fig. 3. NOTE: *Evaluate any pulmonary artery or aortic obstruction if suspected. When position is confirmed the device is released. Take care not to leave the stiff end of the cable against the roof of the MPA in the RVOT.*

Postcatheterization Care

These are usually out-patient procedures. Pro-phylactic antibiotics are routinely administered. Observation is for 4–6 hr in the recovery room (depending on access). A CXR confirms device position and establishes a baseline if a CXR is performed in the future.

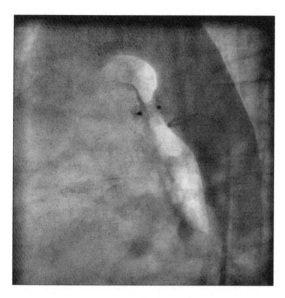

Fig. 3 Angiogram following delivery of an Amplatzer PDA occluder

Results and Complications

Embolization can occur, and is more common with coils, usually to the pulmonary arteries. Incomplete closure is more common when using coils in large PDAs and may rarely be complicated by hemolysis. Left pulmonary artery obstruction can occur with either coils or ADOs and should be evaluated if suspected, particularly in small patients or with large PDAs requiring large devices or multiple coils. Acute closure rates with the ADO are ~70%, with complete occlusion in ~90–95% the following day and >97% by 1 year (1).

Reference

1. Pass RH, Hijazi Z, Hsu DT, Lewis V, Hellenbrand WE. Multicenter USA amplatzer patent ductus arteriosus occlusion device trial. *J Am Coll Cardiol* 2004;44:513–19.

Review Article

Grifka RG. Transcatheter closure of the patent ductus arteriosus. *Cath Card Intv* 2004;61:554–570.

Creating Atrial Septal Defects

Balloon Atrial Septostomy

Since the first report by Rashkind and Miller of a BAS for transposition more than three decades ago, few modifications have occurred in the technique (1). This can be life-saving procedure, equally likely to occur in the middle of the night as it is during the daylight hours. The most common indication for a BAS is D-transposition of the great arteries (dTGA), although rare additional cases do occur.

The intent of the BAS is to create a "tear" in the septum primum flap of the fossa ovalis, thus allow mixing of blood at the atrial level. This can be an intensely satisfying experience because systemic arterial saturations may improve quickly after a successful BAS. Fortunately, the atrial septum in children with dTGA is normally thin, allowing the technique of the BAS to be employed successfully the majority of the time. This is not the case in patients with HLHS and a restrictive atrial septum (see section HLHS with Restrictive Atrial Septum) who require a somewhat more complex and technically difficult procedure.

Precatheterization Considerations and Case Planning

As noted above, usually these are patients with dTGA and a restrictive atrial communication. Review the echo. Be sure you are confident about the cardiac and coronary anatomy. NOTE: *Technically the procedure can be more difficult with juxtaposed appendages or a dilated coronary sinus from an LSVC connection.*

There are two important variables to consider as you quickly plan your case: *where* (catheterization lab vs. ICU) and *how* (umbilical vs. femoral) to do it. Different operators have different preferences, so you can start by asking, but in general:

Advantages of the Catheterization Lab

- If the coronary anatomy is unclear by echo, angiography may be necessary.
- If you want to use umbilical access and you are unable to traverse the liver, fluoroscopy and contrast is required to avoid damage through a tortuous ductus venosus if present.

Advantages of ICU

- Can be done in the ICU at the bedside and no transport is required.
- Quick!

Advantages of Umbilical Access

- Avoids using the groin! Thus, there is no risk of femoral / iliac vein occlusion. If the patient has TGA / VSD / PS and is likely to get an RV-PA homograft (Rastelli), the patient will require catheterization procedures in the future and you may want to consider using an umbilical approach.

L. Bergersen et al. (eds.), *Congenital Heart Disease*,
DOI 10.1007/978-0-387-77292-9_20, © Springer Science+Business Media, LLC 2009

- Patients may already have umbilical venous access prior to procedure with a catheter positioned in the right or left atrium.

Advantages of Femoral Access

- No problems with the ductus venosus being closed or vessel tortuosity.
- Perhaps easier if you are doing an Echo-guided technique because the echocardiographer has more available views to image from, i.e., subxyphoid.

Equipment

We advocate the preparation and maintenance of "Septostomy Kits" that are readily available for these cases which can occur at nearly any time or any place. The following equipment should be considered:

- Septostomy balloon(s)
- Brown 19 G needles
- Micropuncture® Kit
- 18 torque wire(s)
- 6 Fr sheath and 7 Fr sheath
- Assorted syringes

We stock two septostomy catheters:

- Miller Atrioseptostomy Catheter® (Edwards Lifesciences, Germany) Although this catheter is 5 Fr, the nonrecessed balloon requires a 7 Fr introducer sheath. There is a locking mechanism for the inflated balloon. The maximum balloon dilation is 4 cc which equals a 19 mm diameter (2 cc = 16 mm and 1 cc = 13 mm). This catheter has a 35 degree "hockey stick" angled tip to help direct catheter across the pre-existing atrial communication. There is no end-hole. This is the most commonly used BAS catheter at Children's Hospital Boston.
- Atrioseptostomy Balloon Catheter (B. Braun Medical, Inc., Bethlehem, PA). This catheter has the advantage of a low-profile balloon; the balloon and catheter only require a 6 Fr introducer sheath. It also has an end-hole so you can track the catheter over wire (you are almost certainly in the catheterization lab doing this). Maximum balloon 2 cc = 14 mm diameter.

There is no intrinsic locking mechanism (but you can use three-way stop-cock).

Procedure and Techniques

Fluoroscopy Guided

When venous access is established and heparin is administered, the preferred balloon septostomy catheter is inserted through the sheath. Most of the time this will be a Miller balloon, with the metal introducer removed. When in the RA the catheter tip is directed left and posterior towards the LA.

Be careful that the catheter is not in the right ventricle (anterior) or coronary sinus (inferior). When the atrial appendages are juxtaposed accessing the LA can be more difficult because the RA appendage is more leftward and posterior than usual. If this is present or position is not certain, particular attention should be made to advance the catheter tip well posterior and into a LPV.

After confirming catheter position in LA, inflate the balloon slowly to ensure its expansion in the LA cavity and not in the pulmonary vein, LA appendage, or mitral valve. Dilute contrast is used to inflate the balloon. While inflating, the balloon is jiggled back and forth to ensure that it is free within the LA and not entrapped. The balloon must have a uniform spherical shape during inflation. When partially inflated, traction on the catheter brings the balloon against the atrial septum and away from the mitral valve. Retract the sheath into the IVC or umbilical vein.

When your balloon is inflated to the desired amount, lock the catheter and withdraw the catheter to the RA with a rapid, short, jerking motion. Do not hold the sheath. Dr. Keane best explains this motion as "a good back-hand in squash." Re-advancing the catheter with clockwise rotation will confirm passage through the atrial septum, as the catheter enters the SVC. When the balloon reaches the RA it is deflated and advanced back into the LA, and repeated 1–3 times with slightly larger balloons (e.g., first 2.5 to 3 cc, second 3 to 4 cc).

An end-hole catheter may then measure the LA-RA mean pressure gradient. The mean pressure gradient should be less than 2–4 mmHg.

Echo-Guided Technique

Ideal for the ICU setting, but even if in the catheterization lab, you can still use echocardiography, especially if the anatomy is somewhat abnormal (2). You can use umbilical or femoral access. If you are in the ICU, remember the course to the RA via the umbilical vein can be tortuous and difficult. If you already have umbilical access it may be worth a try, but do not waste time if the child is unwell. Also remember, if the child is desaturated (usual) you may have difficulty being sure that you are in a femoral vein.

Use your equipment! Usually you can easily confirm that the wire is in the IVC, SVC, or RA with echo. Do this *prior* to placing a 7 Fr sheath. If the 7 Fr sheath does not pass easily, put in a smaller sheath (3 Fr) and transducer pressure to confirm IVC position. We administer heparin after access is obtained. Place the catheter in the sheath and gently into the heart. Marking on the shaft of the catheter will help you know when echo should be "seeing" the catheter in the heart. It should go almost straight into the LA if angled correctly. Using saline in the balloon, gently inflate the balloon in the LA. Be sure the balloon is not interfering with the mitral valve and that you are in the LA and not a pulmonary vein. Pull the balloon against the atrial septum, then "jerk" the balloon across the septum as previously described. When you are in the RA quickly deflate the balloon and allow the echocardiographer to measure defect size. Hopefully you will see an expected change in the saturations! Repeat as necessary.

Postcatheterization Care

These patients usually will not be going anywhere until surgery. An echocardiogram should confirm the size of the defect and gradient (before you pull sheaths) and should confirm that there is no effusion or damage to the heart.

Results and Complications

Complications of BAS in the newborn period are very rare in the modern era. Rarely an attempt at a bedside BAS will fail due to an inability to pass the catheter through a restrictive or unfavorable PFO and will need to be performed in the catheterization lab. There exist case reports of pulmonary vein, atrial, or hepatic lacerations. BAS has been identified as a risk factor for preoperative CVA in infants with dTGA, but it is unclear if this is procedure or physiology-related (3).

Needle Atrial Transseptal Puncture (Brockenbrough) Technique

Although atrial transseptal approaches were initially described independently by Cope and Ross in 1959, modification by Brockenbrough in 1960 paved the way for more extensive utilization in adults, and subsequently children (4). Further and seemingly innumerable modifications of the technique have occurred, but the general principle remains the same and the procedure can be done safely if intimate knowledge is maintained with the materials and anatomy at play.

Equipment

To perform a Brockenbrough you will need to prepare the following equipment:

- A long sheath of appropriate size and length.
- A transseptal needle.
  - Most come in short [pediatric, ~56 cm] or long [adult, ~71 cm] sizes.
  - Taper from proximal (18–19 g) to distal (21–22 g).
  - A stylet to prevent damage to dilator/sheath during advancement.
  - Needle direction indicator, usually an arrow, near the hub that denotes the direction of curve of the needle.
  - May be included stopcocks.
- If the sheath does not have a side-arm adapter, then prepare a catheter of your choice with a side arm on it to go into the sheath when the dilator is removed.
- A small (3- or 5-cc) syringe with contrast.
- Appropriate wires (see below).

Technique

The Brockenbrough techinque is performed in order to gain access to the LA for the purpose of hemodynamic evaluation and / or intervention. Before reaching for your transseptal needle, first make sure you need it! "Probe-patent" atrial defects (PFOs, etc.) are not uncommon, so just because the precatheterization echo could not see it does not mean it is not there. A multipurpose catheter (Multi) is probably the best catheter for probing the atrial septum in older children and adults. It can also be done with a wedge catheter (balloon down) and the stiff-end of a straight wire bent like a hockey stick and advanced up to, but not beyond, the tip of the catheter. In infants and children with small RAs, Berenstein, Bentson, or JR catheters sometimes offer a better approach. Knowledge of normal atrial anatomy is essential.

The basic technique is as follows:

1. Place a wire of appropriate diameter and length into the SVC.
2. Take your catheters (and old sheath) out over the wire and advance your long sheath and dilator (from the kit or otherwise) over the wire and into the SVC. Remove the wire, but leave the dilator in place.
3. We recommend removing the stylet from the needle, placing a 3-cc syringe with contrast on the back of the transseptal needle, and flushing the needle outside the body. Be aware that some transseptal needles have stopcocks. An alternative approach is to attach a pressure transducer to the needle after the needle is advanced to the end of the sheath and the stylet is removed. The goal of either is to be able to quickly confirm your position.
4. Place the transseptal needle through the dilator. You may need to withdraw the dilator a few millimeters in order get the needle into the dilator without undue force. When the needle is in a few centimeters, advance the dilator into the sheath. NOTE: *The "ruler" on the dilator indicates the distance of the dilator tip from the end of the sheath.*
5. Slowly and gently advance the needle up through the dilator / sheath until just shy of the distal end. (Doing this under fluoroscopy will lessen the chances of puncturing through the wall of the dilator and sheath and into the body.)
6. Inject a small amount of contrast. It should flow freely and be easily seen.
7. This is a two-handed technique. The left hand holds a constant relationship between the needle and dilator. The right hand steers via the needle direction indicator and is available to inject contrast.
8. The unit (needle / dilator / sheath) is pulled back under constant fluoroscopic visualization with the whole unit pointed posterior and leftward (Figure 1). The camera angles under which this is done vary from place to place. With a biplane lab, PA and lateral are fine. Left anterior oblique is common as well.
9. The unit (needle / dilator / sheath) will, in the usual situation, "jump" as it reaches the fossa ovalis (usually about two-thirds of the way down the RA silhouette). Continue to bring it down slightly further. Advancement as soon as it jumps will often be quite high with the needle entering the LA near the "roof."
10. Place the tip of the needle just at the tip of the dilator.
11. At this point injection of a small amount of contrast through the needle will stain the septum. If you are convinced of appropriate position, a short jab with a smooth but forceful advancement of the needle should puncture the septum and cross into the LA. Take care not to jab and recoil, in which case you may puncture the septum but fall back to the RA. Injection of contrast will confirm position if your needle tip is in the LA; see Figure 1.
12. *Without moving the needle,* advance the dilator and sheath over the needle and into the LA using steady forward pressure and some rotation. When the sheath is securely in position, withdraw the needle only first to the RA and then the dilator, to avoid buckling of the sheath in the LA. Now you are ready.

Tips:

- An arterial catheter in the ascending aorta will mark the position of the aortic root. Stay posterior to this.
- Levophase of a PA angiogram will highlight the LA for direct visualization.

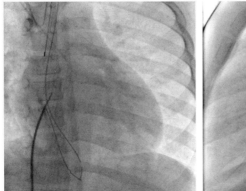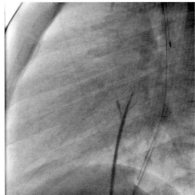

Fig. 1 Transeptal needle puncture

- Constant control of the (needle / dilator / sheath) unit is required and one should never let go or relax control as this will almost always result in malposition.
- With repeated manipulation the degree of agreement between the actual needle curve and the needle curve indicator may vary. Always watch the monitors!
- If you cannot advance the sheath, advance just the dilator; if you can do that, place a 0.014″ wire through the needle into a pulmonary vein. With this in place you can usually advance a coronary balloon and dilate the septum, then advance your sheath over the balloon as it is deflated.
- At all times respect the LA and avoid injection of air or anything else!
- Some operators will not administer heparin until after successful transseptal access has been achieved (in case the heart is punctured). If this is the practice, do not forget to give the heparin as soon as you are there!
- Patients with LA hypertension will often have "bowing" of the atrial septum, and the "jump" into the fossa ovalis will often be subtle or absent. Know your landmarks.
- Beware of conditions that affect the usual anatomic orientations, including thoracic deformities (scoliosis, etc.), dilated aortic roots, LA hypertension or very dilated atria, and HLHS (very small LAs). Consider a PA angiogram in these patients.

- The approach from the left groin is different from the right and may require modification of the needle angle.
- A surgical (patched) atrial septum is frequently more difficult to cross. A slight bend (exaggerating the native transseptal needle curve) several centimeters back from the needle tip will allow a more perpendicular application of force and lessen the odds of "sliding up the septum." Do not sacrifice the structural integrity of the needle to do this!

HLHS with Restrictive Atrial Septum

The atrial septum in infants with HLHS can be very thick, and if restrictive these newborns become critically ill. In this situation an effective BAS is almost never possible, because the septum primum is not only thick but also can have abnormal attachments that may be dangerous to the child's health. Therefore, the usual approach at Children's Hospital Boston is to create a separate defect in the atrial septum by Brockenbrough puncture or radiofrequency wire perforation. The atrial defect is then dilated by short, high-pressure balloons and then usually stented. The LA in these patients is typically very small and makes this procedure challenging.

Precatheterization Considerations and Case Planning

Newborns with HLHS and a restrictive or intact atrial septum are usually very sick. In fact, there are only a handful of situations when a newborn with congenital heart disease needs to come urgently to the catheterization lab from the delivery room—*this is one*. As such, advance notice is always desirable, and thanks to prenatal echocardiography this is often the case. The work-up is straightforward, particularly if there is a recent and reliable prenatal echocardiogram. A limited echocardiogram can be performed after birth, but after the diagnosis is confirmed either echocardiographically or clinically the infant should be transferred to the catheterization lab without delay.

Procedure and Techniques

This procedure needs to be performed quickly and precisely. Only experienced fellows should be scrubbed at these cases. The neonate is prepped and draped quickly and femoral access is obtained, preferably from the right. Arterial access is nice but should not delay decompression of the atrial septum. Occasionally there is an existing defect that is in a reasonable position but is simply too small. In this case it is often possible to pass a 0.014″ wire through the defect and into the LA or pulmonary vein. The remainder of the technique is similar to that described below for the intact atrial septum.

Brockenbrough Technique

In the situation of an intact atrial septum or an unfavorable or inaccessible restrictive defect you need to make your own. Using a modified Brockenbrough technique the LA is entered with the needle. There is no fossa ovalis in these patients, so the puncture site on the atrial septum is identified without the usual drag-down technique.

After a stain is made in the septum, work quickly because you can utilize this stain, while the visible location helps guide stent placement. Remember, there is often little room between the thick atrial septum (now displaced by the needle) and the posterior wall of the LA.

When the needle is in the LA it is often quite difficult to pass the dilator, and always difficult, if not close to impossible, to pass the long sheath. Therefore, when you have the needle through, remove the syringe from the back of the needle and advance a 0.014 wire through the needle into a stable (all things being relative) position in the LA (appendage, pulmonary vein, or looped within the LA).

You should be able to advance at least the dilator into the LA. If the sheath will not advance beyond the septum the dilator can be removed over the wire (*do not lose wire position!*) and a coronary balloon may be passed over the wire and dilated across the atrial septum. As the balloon is deflated the sheath can be passed over the balloon into the LA Fig. 2. With stable sheath position, the desired stent (short and about 5 mm in diameter, Fig. 3) can be placed across the septum and dilated to the desired degree, often based on measurement of the residual gradient across the septum (5 mmHg is a reasonable stopping point, but this depends on many things).

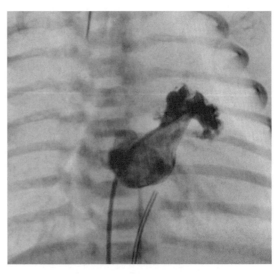

Fig. 2 LA angiogram restrictive septum

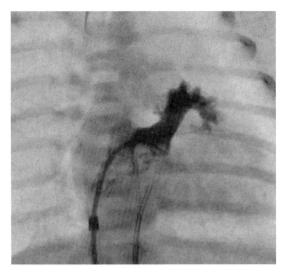

Fig. 3 Stented atrial septum

Radiofrequency Perforation

An alternative to the Brockenbrough technique is the use of an RFCA to "burn" across the atrial septum. For this technique, use a stiff-shaped catheter positioned against the atrial septum. Trans-thoracic echo can be helpful in guiding this intervention. Subsequent procedural details are similar to that above.

Postcatheterization Care

Echocardiography should be performed to confirm the size of the tear / communication, trans-septal gradient, and to ensure there is no significant pericardial effusion related to unsuspected tears of the atrial wall or pulmonary veins. These patients go to the ICU to recover and will likely get the necessary imaging (echo, CXR), laboratory studies (Hct), and antibiotics as a part of their routine care. Heparin is generally given until the stent is removed at surgery.

Results and Complications

These patients are critically ill to begin with and have a poor prognosis. They start their lives facing the risks of this procedure which include tears or perforations of the atrial wall / appendage, pulmonary vein, or inferior vena cava, damage to the atrio-ventricular valves, and atrial and ventricular arrhythmias. Balloon rupture is rare but should be anticipated, and care should be taken to avoid air embolism. Stent malposition can occur but can usually be managed either by telescoping stents or stent reposition.

References

1. Rashkind WJ, Miller WW. Creation of an atrial septal defect without thoracotomy: a palliative approach to complete transposition of the great vessels. *J Am Med Assoc* 1966;196:991–992.
2. Allan LD, Sharland GK. The echocardiographic diagnosis of totally anomalous pulmonary venous connection in the fetus. *Heart* 2001;85:433–437.
3. McQuillen PS, Hamrick SE, Perez MJ et al. Balloon atrial septostomy is associated with preoperative stroke in neonates with transposition of the great arteries. *Circulation.* 2006;113:280–285.
4. Duff DF, Mullins CE. Transseptal left heart catheterization in infants and children. *Catheterization and Cardiovascular Diagnosis.* 1978;4:213–223.

Pericardiocentesis

Introduction

The indications for removal of fluid from the pericardial space fall into two categories: diagnostic and therapeutic. Most diagnostic pericardiocenteses occur in the context of chronic effusions, to assess for viral or bacterial infection, neoplasia, storage disease, or a connective tissue disorder. Therapeutic "taps" may be required in either elective or emergent circumstances. The former will include patients with recurrent, large-volume pericardial effusions, with a myriad of causes, including post-pericardiotomy syndrome, neoplasia, disorders of lymphatic drainage, and idiopathic effusions. Most of the emergent procedures are the result of misadventures in the catheterization lab or in hemodynamically compromised postoperative patients.

Precatheterization Considerations and Case Planning

Most of these cases are "add-ons"—patients who urgently or semi-urgently require this procedure. The work-up will range from quite straightforward, if they have no structural heart disease, to quite complex. Either way, a full knowledge of their history and hemodynamic status is imperative. These patients will have had, in nearly all nonemergent cases, an echocardiogram. Echocardiography can demonstrate the size and location of the effusion, both of which are important if you plan to drain it, and may describe many apparent hemodynamic abnormalities associated with elevated intracardiac pressure. However, remember that the decision to drain the fluid is a clinical one, and one that incorporates more than just the echo. Similarly, tamponade is a clinical diagnosis.

Cardiac catheterization is not routinely performed for isolated pericardial effusions. However, you should be familiar with the pathophysiology at play. A brief discussion on hemodynamic findings in pericardial disease can be found in the hemodynamics chapter in Part I.

Equipment

- 8 Fr Periocardiocentesis Set (Cook, Inc., Bloomington, IN) which includes an 18 gauge pink introducer needle, J-tipped 0.038 wire, 8 Fr dilator, 8 Fr pigtail catheter, and ThoraSeal™ connector. A 5 or 6 Fr pigtail and 0.035 wire can be used for infants.
- Large (30 and / or 60 cc) Luer Lock syringes and three-way stop-cock.
- Containers for samples to be sent to lab for culture, cell count, cytology, chemistry, etc.
- Pleuravac® collection container.

Procedure and Techniques

It is mandatory to have echocardiography and / or fluoroscopy to guide the placement of the needle and catheter unless the patient is in extremis. We do not practice the use of EKG monitoring of the needle with an alligator clip, but do watch for ectopy on the surface EKG. If you are not in a rush, a brief stored fluoroscopic PA image can be performed prior to catheter placement and repeated at the end.

The patient is prepped and draped in the usual fashion. In some cases positioning the patient

L. Bergersen et al. (eds.), *Congenital Heart Disease*,
DOI 10.1007/978-0-387-77292-9_21, © Springer Science+Business Media, LLC 2009

sitting somewhat upright can be helpful. Because you always use echo, you can allow the echocardiographer to locate the largest, most easily accessible pocket of fluid. *Again, you are looking for the largest most easily accessible pocket of fluid.* This is often, but not always, best accessed from the subxiphoid region. However, if the largest amount of fluid is best accessed through the thorax, then the best intercostal space (largest amount of fluid closest to the chest wall) should be sought.

Know your anatomy (intercostal, internal mammary and coronary vessels, lung, etc.), and positions other than subxiphoid that can be used safely. At this point, the person performing the procedure should take the transducer (in a sterile sleeve) and assess the angle of the probe that identifies the best trajectory (shortest distance, straight shot). This is the angle of your needle. Memorize it, and note the distance from skin to fluid to heart. Apply topical anesthetic, give it time to work, and grab the needle. Re-echo if you need confirmation of your approach.

The percutaneous needle, with or without a small syringe attached to it and with no Luer Lock, is inserted through the skin in the direction outlined by the echo findings. If using a syringe gentle negative pressure is applied to the syringe. Fluid should be encountered within 1 cm of the depth estimated by echo. If not, withdraw to the skin, redirect slightly and try again. Fellows generally insert the needle at too steep of an angle. Entrance into the pericardial space is identified by the free flow of fluid into the syringe. Chronic effusion fluid will usually be blood tinged, but frank blood may indicate that you have entered the heart. If you are concerned that you may have entered the ventricle, advance a soft wire through the needle and see where it goes by fluoroscopy and / or echo. Also, pericardial fluid will not clot as readily and will soak into a piece of gauze, rather than remaining on top of it.

When you are confident that the needle tip is in the pericardial space, remove the syringe and place the guide wire through the hub. The wire should travel posterior to the heart on lateral fluoroscopy imaging. It should be easy to advance. When the position is confirmed, remove the needle, leaving the wire in place. Place a nick in the skin with a scalpel. Dilate the entry site and pericardium with a dilator. Place the pigtail catheter over the wire and advance into the pericardial space. Cover the end with the stopcock. The catheter can be sewn in place if drainage is to continue after the procedure. Remove fluid with large syringes and then hook up to the Thora-Seal using the included connector.

Emergent Pericardiocentesis

Emergency situations result in modification of the above procedure in several key elements:

- The patient will often be moving (from CPR, etc.).
- You have to be faster, often with less help from imaging modalities such as echo.
- You may need to do a "blind" needle insertion, with the needle inserted 1–2 cm below the xiphoid process at an angle of 25–45 degrees to the horizontal plane, in the direction of the left shoulder.
- You may want to remove some fluid via the needle, before placing the pigtail, in order to get a rapid improvement in hemodynamic status. Due to compliance of the pericardium, you need to remove relatively little fluid in order to improve tamponade physiology.
- If there is a persistent leak, you may be back to the starting level in pretty short order.
- Sterile technique may be suboptimal; remember to get some antibiotics on board as soon as possible.
- If you do not have a pigtail kit, you can use any catheter! Get into the pericardial space and start draining fluid; a catheter with multiple side-holes such as a pig tail will be most efficient.
- You can even use a 16 or 18 gauge Angiocath[TM] in a dire emergency. When fluid is encountered, hook up a T-connector piece and a three-way stop cock and start sucking out fluid. Most operators recommend removing the needle from the Angiocath, although some operators leave it in when there is a large effusion to prevent collapse of the Angiocath tubing. This can be very dangerous, and even fatal, if the needle is left up against the beating heart, since a linear cardiac tear can produce massive hemopericardium. It is imperative that you maintain the relation of the catheter to the skin to avoid losing position. This set-up can be switched out when the emergency subsides.

Postcatheterization Care

In most cases the pigtail pericardial drain is left in place and is secured and draped in a sterile manner. Prophylactic antibiotics are not routinely administered in all cases. A postprocedural CXR (in two views) is performed to document cardiac silhouette size and catheter position. The decision to remove the catheter, which can be done at the bedside, is, again, a clinical one.

Results and Complications

Injury to the coronary artery is one of the most serious complications. This is best avoided by using echocardiography and fluoroscopy, and possibly by directing the needle posterior and toward the left shoulder when using a subxiphoid approach. Other approaches can be more risky. Intraventricular puncture is also a possibility, but tends to be less problematic, as long as it is recognized before the dilator is placed. Ventricular laceration has occurred. Pneumothoraces generally result from inserting the needle in a greater depth than necessary and by aiming too laterally.

Additional Reading

Lang P. Other catheterization laboratory techniques and interventions. In: *Diagnostic and Interventional Catheterization in Congenital Heart Disease*, 2nd ed. Kluwer Academic Publishers, Norwell, MA, 2000.

Endomyocardial Biopsy

Introduction

The most common indication for an endomyocardial biopsy (EMB) is surveillance for post–heart transplant cellular rejection. Another frequent indication is in idiopathic cardiomyopathies, as a guide for therapy (myocarditis vs. cardiomyopathy) or for prognostic purposes (cardiomyopathy, glycogen storage disease, metabolic disorders).

Precatheterization Considerations and Case Planning

In patients after transplant it is important to know the following details about the history:

- Pretransplant diagnosis (cardiomyopathy vs. complex congenital heart disease).
- Pretransplant anatomic anomalies (pulmonary artery, pulmonary vein, systemic venous stenoses, coarctation, or collateral vessels).
- Posttransplant anatomic anomalies (anastomotic obstructions: SVC, IVC, MPA, and aAo).
- Known vessel occlusion (documented or suspected occlusions, history of ECMO cannulation, and sites of vessel reconstruction).
- Hemodynamic data from the previous several biopsy procedures.
- Requirements for sedation/anesthesia.

Equipment

Although a variety of bioptomes are available we use the 5 Fr SparrowHawk® (ATC Technologies, Inc., Woburn MA); 50 cm for children and adults from the IJV or SCV approach, and 105 cm for adolescents and adults from the femoral venous approach. We perform these cases with a Cook 5 Fr 45 cm long sheath for IJV or SCV access in all patients, or groin access in small children, and a Cook 6 Fr 85 cm long sheath for femoral vein access in older children and adults; however, other types of sheaths may be used. Additional equipment includes a brown needle (18 g), transducer, an 18″ torque wire, 6 Fr short dilator, wedge catheter and (if appropriate) pigtail catheter and coronary arteriography catheters.

Procedure and Techniques

Vascular Access

We usually access via the femoral or subclavian veins in posttransplant patients <15 kg (< 2 years old). This is primarily due to vessel size, and the implications of thrombosis developing with frequent biopsies in the initial posttransplant period. We usually transition to the RIJV or SCV at 2–3 years of age. The main advantage for IJV or SCV access is that the patient can ambulate immediately after the procedure. However, the IJV is not used if the contralateral IJV is occluded. The femoral vein is used when access to the femoral artery is planned as part of the procedure. And if additional interventions are planned, the sheath size and approach to the site of intervention are taken into consideration.

Hemodynamics

Right-sided hemodynamics in room air include PA and/or SVC saturation and the following

L. Bergersen et al. (eds.), *Congenital Heart Disease*,
DOI 10.1007/978-0-387-77292-9_22, © Springer Science+Business Media, LLC 2009

pressures: PCW, PA, RV, RA, and SVC or IVC. Abnormal data should be further studied with appropriate hemodynamic measurements or angiography.

Biopsies in patients with cardiomyopathies are usually only one part of a complete pretransplant evaluation that will determine whether a patient is a candidate for heart transplantation. In these cases you must identify any anatomic lesions or hemodynamic findings in which an intervention or changes in medical management strategy might improve the clinical situation and obviate or delay the need for transplant. Further, you should obtain an accurate measurement of the pulmonary vascular resistance at the baseline, and if indicated reassess on oxygen and nitric therapy. Make sure if a respiratory or metabolic acidosis is present that it is corrected so that the PVR is not overestimated.

Preparing the Sheath

The long sheath and bioptome should be formed, prior to insertion in the patient, such that the sheath tip and bioptome are directed toward the RV septum (1). The long sheaths are made with a 70° curve 1–2 cm from the end of the sheath. Create a 90° angle, starting 3–8 cm from the tip of the sheath (depending on the size of the patient) so that after it is in the body this curve will occur in the RA, directing the sheath into the RV. Next, bend the distal portion of the sheath perpendicular to this curve to point the sheath posterior to the RV septum. Note that this curve will be a mirror image if approaching from above (IJV) or below (femoral vein). The curves are best made by gently and smoothly stripping the sheath / dilator over your thumb. The final shape will direct the sheath tip rightward through the tricuspid valve, inferiorly

toward the RV apex and posterior toward the ventricular septum, Figure 1.

After the sheath is in position, examine the position of the sheath within the RV by fluoroscopy, or less commonly inject contrast through the sheath to delineate RV anatomy. Problems with the sheath position are usually overcome by appropriately bending the bioptome. In all cases formable bioptomes must be prebent because the sheath will lose its shape with a stiff bioptome inside. The bioptome is formed in a similar manner to that described for the sheath, with a bend directing the bioptome across the tricuspid valve (3–8 cm away from the forceps) and into the RV apex and another bend (close to the forceps) directing the tip posterior to the RV septum.

With the bioptome advanced to the end of the sheath, turn the handle counterclockwise (from IJV or SCV approaches) or clockwise (from femoral vein approach) to further direct the bioptome posteriorly. NOTE: *If you are unsure of the bends in the equipment you have created, try this motion outside the body to assure the equipment will be directed posterior towards the septum.*

Open the jaws while the bioptome is within the sheath, then advance the bioptome out of the sheath. As you gently advance the bioptome you should see the bioptome open and the sheath start to recess and / or the bioptome shaft start to bend. This tells you that the tip of the bioptome is against the myocardium. Close the jaws, readvance the sheath while gently pulling back on the bioptome. (NOTE: *Particularly in small children, the bioptome does not need to be advanced far to appose myocardium. Start without a lot of forward tension on the bioptome and see if you get a piece (you may be surprised); if unsuccessful, then push forward more next time.*) Remove the bioptome, holding the jaws shut.

The specimen is placed in a container and repeat biopsies are obtained. Between each biopsy the long sheath should be flushed (to ensure that it is not up against myocardium and to clear the sheath of air). The bioptome may need to be re-bent slightly to direct the forceps to a different site along the septum. Five pieces (≥1 mm) are collected from the RV septum in posttransplant patients and reviewed under light microscopy for cellular rejection. Recently, additional tests are considered such

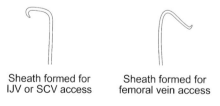

Sheath formed for   Sheath formed for
IJV or SCV access   femoral vein access

Fig. 1 Shaped sheath for RV biopsy

as C4d staining for humoral rejection. Biopsies from *pretransplant patients* are processed in several ways: electron microscopy, light microscopy, and freezing / saving.

Postcatheterization Care

Fluoroscopy should be considered following access from the SCV, to check for hemo- or pneumothorax, prior to the patient leaving the catheterization lab. Following removal of catheters from the IJV or SCV the patient should be placed at an incline to avoid bleeding or hematoma. After removal of catheters from the femoral vein the patient should remain supine for at least 3 hr if heparin was not given. If heparin was given, the patient is chronically anticoagulated, or arterial access was obtained, the patient should remain supine for 6 hr. A postcatheterization hematocrit is not generally obtained.

Results and Complications

Myocardial perforation, pneumothorax, sustained arrhythmias, unresolved heart block, tricuspid valve damage, air and clot emboli, interventricular septal perforation, pericardial tamponade, and puncture of the carotid artery are all potential but rare and unusual complications of this procedure. Risk of perforation is highest among patients with suspected myocarditis and dilated cardiomyopathy (2).

References

1. Hauptman PJ, Gass A, Cohen M et al. Endomyocardial biopsy: advantages of adding a posterior bend to the bioptome. *Cathet Cardiovasc Diagn* 1992;27: 228–229.
2. Pophal SG, Sigfusson G, Booth KL et al. Complications of endomyocardial biopsy in children. *J Am Coll Cardiol* 1999;34(7):2105–2110.

Coronary Angiography

Coronary Arteries in Congenital and Acquired Heart Disease

Proximal coronary anatomy can usually be well documented by 2D echo and color flow imaging. CT angiography and even MRI are increasingly common, although not in most pediatric centers yet. There remain, however, situations where conventional coronary angiography is useful.

Among the acquired lesions, coronary angiography is performed regularly following orthotopic heart transplant, looking for signs of coronary artery disease related to chronic rejection. Occasionally imaging of coronary aneurysms and stenosis is required in patients with Kawasaki disease, especially in high-risk patients with giant aneurysms, abnormal exercise testing, or clinical symptoms. Coronary artery fistulae (congenital or acquired) usually can be seen by CT, but assessing the feasibility of trans-catheter closure usually requires conventional angiography (and you can close it while you are there).

There are seemingly innumerable congenital coronary variations, normal and otherwise, in the origin and course of the coronary arteries in congenital heart disease. In some cases the variation is the essence of the malformation itself, as is the case with isolated anomalous connection of the left coronary artery to the pulmonary artery (ALCAPA). In other cases, coronary variations are of surgical importance, as in D-transposition of the great arteries or pulmonary atresia with intact ventricular septum. The distinction is some-what artificial, but solid knowledge of normal and abnormal coronary circulations and their surgical importance are crucial to those performing coronary angiography. Also important is proficiency with the means by which to safely image the coronary arteries, because even the smallest errors of technique can quickly have significant consequences.

While a detailed account of all coronary artery abnormalities in congenital heart disease is well beyond the scope of this manual, this chapter will briefly discuss techniques common to identifying the more frequent abnormalities.

Normal Coronary Arteries

In the normal heart the right and left coronary arteries arise from the respective sinuses, typically midway between the aortic valve commissures and two-thirds of the distance from the annulus to the sino-tubular junction. Separate ostia of the conus branch and left circumflex are considered normal variants.

- In its proximal course, the *left main coronary artery* (LCA) lies between the left atrium and pulmonary trunk, and is covered by the left atrial appendage. It bifurcates into the *left anterior descending* (LAD) and left *circumflex* arteries in two-thirds of individuals and tri-furcates into these and a third intermediate artery in the other one-third. In ~1% of patients, the circumflex and LAD arise from separate orifices from the left coronary sinus. This occurs more frequently in patients with bi-commissural aortic valves. Epicardial branches from the LAD are called *diagonals*, and are numbered sequentially as they arise. Branches that supply the interventricular septum are called *septal perforators*. A short LCA is associated with left dominance.

L. Bergersen et al. (eds.), *Congenital Heart Disease*,
DOI 10.1007/978-0-387-77292-9_23, © Springer Science+Business Media, LLC 2009

- The LAD travels in the anterior interventricular groove, wraps around the apex, and travels a variable distance in the posterior interventricular groove. Together with its diagonals and septal perforators the LAD typically supplies the anteroseptal and anterolateral LV walls, the anterolateral papillary muscle and the LV apex. Myocardial bridging can be observed in up to 10% of adults and produce systolic narrowing in up to 2%. The prognosis is usually benign.

- The left *circumflex* coronary artery (Circ) travels in the left AV groove, the branches of which are called obtuse marginals. The Circ typically supplies the lateral LV free wall, the anterolateral papillary muscle. In about 10–15% of patients, the Circ also gives rise to the *posterior descending artery* (PDA), constituting left coronary dominance, which supplies the inferoseptal wall of the LV and the posteromedial papillary muscle. In about 20% of hearts the PDA is supplied by both the right and left circumflex coronary arteries, in so-called *shared dominance*.

- The *right coronary artery* (RCA) travels between the pulmonary trunk and the right atrium, covered by the right atrial appendage. In about 60% of hearts the first branch of the RCA is the *conus coronary artery*, which supplies the right ventricular outflow tract. In the other 40% of hearts the conus coronary arises separately from the right aortic sinus. *Marginal branches* include several small vessels and a prominent *acute marginal*. The RCA gives rise to both the PDA and posterolateral branches in about 70% of hearts. In such a situation, these vessels supply not only the RV free wall, but also the LV inferoseptal wall and posteromedial papillary muscle.

- *Coronary supply of the conduction system:* The sinus node is supplied by the RCA in 60% of hearts and the Circ in 40%. The AV node is supplied by the dominant coronary artery (RCA in 90% of hearts). The His bundles are supplied dually by the first septal perforator and the AV node artery. The right and left bundles are usually supplied by septal perforators of the LAD and PDA, respectively.

- The coronary veins usually parallel the arteries. The great cardiac vein travels with the LAD and then goes along the left AV groove, becoming the coronary sinus posteriorly. Several other large veins drain into the CS, including the left marginal vein, the middle cardiac vein (posterior interventricular groove), and small cardiac vein (right AV groove). The normal CS drains into the inferior and posterior right atrium. The anterior RV veins drain directly into the RA.

Equipment

In some situations a simple ascending aortogram performed through a pigtail catheter or other angiographic catheter will suffice in providing the necessary anatomic information. In other situations, selective coronary angiography is required. For the latter, a familiar but not dogged adherence to the usual armament of coronary catheters (chiefly, Judkins and Amplatz catheters) is necessary. (Refer to the catheters and wires chapter in Part I.)

A coronary manifold system is preferable to directly injecting contrast through the end of a catheter in the coronary artery. This closed system allows the operator to quickly alternate between pressure measurement, flush, and contrast manipulation, and minimizes the risks of air emboli and unrecognized coronary occlusion by the catheter. It should go without mention that most catheter exchanges should be performed over a wire (preferably J wire), and all catheters should be flushed prior to use.

With normal coronary arteries, if the correct catheter is chosen the catheter should almost literally fall into the coronary orifice. In other situations, small and gentle catheter manipulations may be required. Any time that you think you may be at or near the coronary orifice you should quickly check pressure. Proximal coronary pressure in a nonobstructed vessel essentially looks like an ascending aortic tracing. If anything other than this is observed you should presume complete or partial coronary occlusion and gently (but quickly) withdraw the catheter. After you have obtained a good position, give a small test injection, adjust your camera angles as needed, and perform your angiography. If you have a good pressure tracing and you need additional angles the catheter can be left in position, the cameras adjusted, and further angiography performed.

Angiographic Projections

The types of projections used will vary significantly, based on the indication for catheterization. In general, selective coronary artery imaging is used when there are questions about the course and caliber of the coronary arteries. In a heart with normal ventricular and arterial relations, there are standard projections that are recommended to image each coronary artery. The goal of all of these is to be in a position that is tangential to the area of interest, thereby lengthening the course of

the coronary artery in that region. Ideally, you should examine more than one view of each region, as stenoses and aneurysms are not always uniform around the circumference of the vessel. However, before demonstrating typical angiographic projections, it is often useful to remember the appearance of normal coronary angiography in straight PA and lateral (Fig. 1 and Fig. 2).

Specific Angiographic Projections

The angles given below generally provide adequate visualization, but low volume hand injections should be performed prior to cine-angiography to allow adjustments of the angles on an individual basis.

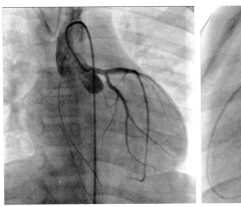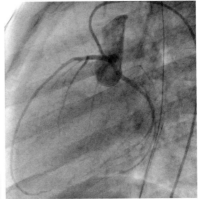

Fig. 1 Left coronary artery angiography

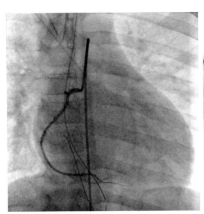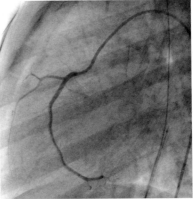

Fig. 2 Right coronary artery angiography

Left Main Coronary Artery

The LCA is often best seen in the "spider view" obtained with the following camera angle: $45° - 60°$ LAO $+ 15° - 25°$ caudal, Fig. 3. The proximal course can also be seen with $15°$ RAO $+ 25°$ caudal angles, Fig. 4.

Left Anterior Descending Artery

The LAD may have to be visualized using several views, due to its length. One of the three best views of the LAD is $15°$ RAO $+ 25°$ caudal, Fig. 4; the entire length of the LAD will be seen well with septal perforators and diagonals clearly delineated. The other nice view is $10°$ RAO $+ 40°$ cranial, Fig. 5. A view similar to the hepatoclavicular view ($45°$ LAO $+ 25° - 35°$ cranial) will elongate the interventricular septum and show the middle and terminal portions of the LAD, Fig. 6.

Left Circumflex Artery

The circumflex is best seen with the RAO and LAO views with caudal angulation, Figs. 3 and 4. LAO with caudal angulation (spider view) will cause the

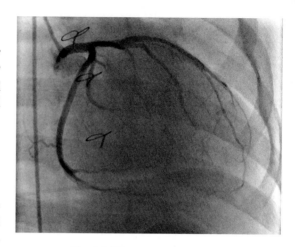

Fig. 4 LCA system, RAO caudal

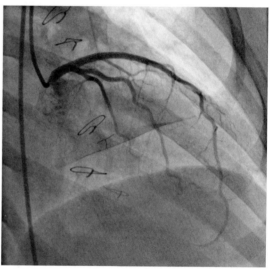

Fig. 5 LCA system, RAO cranial

beam to look up the barrel of the left ventricle, outlining the course around the posterior AV groove.

Right Coronary Artery

The proximal RCA is best seen in either the LAO or straight lateral projections. To lengthen the course of the mid-RCA, use the RAO projection.

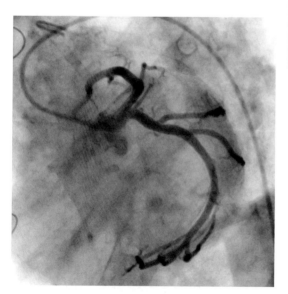

Fig. 3 LCA system, LAO caudal

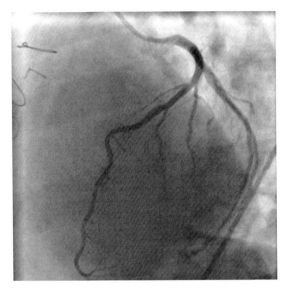

Fig. 6 LCA system, LAO cranial

The posterior descending is best seen with 30° LAO + 30°–45° cranial angulation.

Typical Sequence of Angiograms

LCA System

- 10° RAO + 40° cranial: excellent of LAD; OK of Cx
- 45° LAO + 25° caudal: excellent of LCA, prox LAD/Cx, good of distal Cx
- 15° RAO + 25° caudal: excellent of LMCA/LAD and Cx
- 45° LAO + 25° cranial: very nice LAD, Cx

RCA System

- AP: nice view of mid-portion RCA
- Lateral: excellent proximal RCA, mid-portion RCA
- 30° RAO: excellent mid-portion RCA
- 30° LAO + 30°–45° cranial: excellent distal RCA/PDA

NOTE: *In a biplane lab by alternating cranial / caudal positions with the AP/lateral cameras you will avoid the cameras interfering with each other.*

Specific Examples

D-Transposition of the Great Arteries (dTGA)

Sufficient coronary detail is usually apparent by echocardiography, but angiography remains important in select cases. Coronary angiography in dTGA is usually performed one of two ways. The first takes advantage of the fact that the aorta arises from the RV, allowing easy access from the central venous system. In this case (either before or after a BAS if required), a Berman catheter is advanced antegrade out the RV to the ascending aorta. From here appropriate balloon inflation will subtotally occlude flow and a power injection will force contrast retrograde, filling the coronary arteries (do not forget to take the balloon down afterward). The best angle for an initial angiogram is usually the "laid back" view. This provides an excellent "on-end" view from the bottom of the great arteries and well characterizes their relation to each other (the PA filling slightly later from the PDA). Adjust the cameras as necessary. The other approach is the usual retrograde approach with either an appropriate ascending aortogram or selective coronary injections.

There is a broad spectrum to coronary variation in dTGA; see Figure 7. The term "usual" is preferred to "normal" (because they are certainly not normal) for the most common situation in which the LCA arises from the leftward and anterior-facing sinus and the RCA arises from the posterior-facing sinus. However, it is better practice to describe the anatomy with more detail, by clearly describing the origin, relationships, and proximal course of the coronary arteries.

Pulmonary Atresia with Intact Ventricular Septum (PA/IVS)

Although other criteria play significant roles, one key element in decision making for patients born with PA/IVS is the presence or absence of right ventricular–dependant coronary circulation (RVDCC). The presence of RVDCC precludes safe RV decompression. Because of the

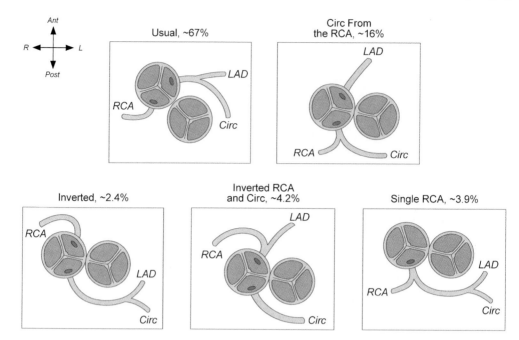

Fig. 7 Coronary anatomy in dTGA (Adapted from Wernovsky et al. Coronary artery anatomy and transposition of the great arteries. *Coronary Artery Dis* 1193;4:148–157, with permission.)

unusual situation in PA/IVS, detailed coronary angiography requires both imaging from the aorta and from the RV.

A common approach is to first enter the RV cavity with an appropriate catheter. This may be a Berman in the situation were the RV cavity permits all the angiographic side-holes of the Berman, a balloon end-hole ("wedge") catheter or a shaped catheter (coronary or otherwise). With the small RV volumes seen in many patients with PA/IVS, often a simple hand injection suffices to detail RV sinusoids and coronary communications as the case may be. Angiography of the aorto-coronary connections and courses should follow. In the most extreme cases there may be no direct communication between the coronary arteries and the aorta (i.e., atresia of the orifices).

The definition of right ventricular coronary dependence has not been unanimously agreed upon. However, it has been shown that:

- RV decompression in the setting of coronary fistulae without stenosis of the origins or distal coronary vessels does not appear to result in death or LV dysfunction, and
- RV decompression in the setting of coronary fistulae and stenosis in both the RCA and LCA/circ systems frequently results in death.

RV decompression in the setting of fistulae and obstruction of a single coronary may carry some risk. It has been the practice at Children's Hospital Boston to decompress the RV in patients with PA/IVS unless there is/are:

- Ventriculo-coronary artery fistulae with severe obstruction of at least two major coronary arteries;
- Complete atresia of the aortic coronary ostia; or
- A significant portion of the LV myocardium appears to be supplied by the RV and is judged to be at risk if RV decompression was performed.

The procedure for trans-catheter pulmonary valve perforation is described in the chapter on PA/IVS.

Anomalous Connection of the Left Coronary Artery and the Pulmonary Artery (ALCAPA)

The straightforward name of this lesion belies the complexity and diversity of anatomy and physiology possible under this heading; and, in actuality, while the LCA is the most common coronary involved in an anomalous connection (preferred over "origin" due to developmental reasons) to a PA, any coronary artery may be so connected. This anomaly usually occurs in isolation although it has been described with a variety of congenital cardiac lesions. The connection to the PA is usually at the facing PA sinus, but can occur to the MPA or either proximal branch PA, and the normally connected coronary artery is usually quite dilated. Selective angiography of the normally connected coronary artery usually shows the anomalously connected coronary filling retrograde via collaterals. An aortogram or selective injection in the left and noncoronary cusps also may be performed.

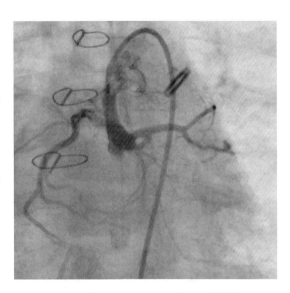

Fig. 8 Coronary angiography in HLHS

Right from the Left, Left from the Right, and Variations

Imbedded in the spectrum of variation of coronary origin and course are those that are abnormal, defined as those occurring in less than 1% of the population, or those that carry some identifiable risk to the patient. The most frequent of these are anomalous origin of the LCA from the right coronary sinus and anomalous origin of the RCA from the left coronary sinus, the former being worse. Identification of these is performed in the usual way, with care taken, understanding that the coronary orifice may be narrowed (slit-like) or eccentrically located within the sinus (this can be diagnosed with IVUS). Selective hand injection in the aortic cusp from which the coronary artery should, but does not, arise may be desirable. Identification of an intramural coronary artery course can be difficult by selective angiography, and may be best characterized by CT angiography which has the advantage of imaging both the contrast-filled arteries and the walls of the great vessels.

Coronaries Through a Stansel or in an Unrepaired HLHS

On occasion, imaging of the coronary arteries following a Stansel anastomosis is required. More rarely, you will need to see them in unrepaired HLHS. The catheters and techniques to do so will greatly depend upon the underlying cardiac malformation and the surgical technique utilized in performance of the anastomosis. In patients with HLHS the native ascending aorta may be quite small, resembling in some situations a "common coronary" itself. In these situations simple injection into the native ascending aorta often provides beautiful anatomic detail, Fig. 8.

Tetralogy of Fallot (ToF)

The most frequent coronary consideration in patients with Tetralogy of Fallot is exclusion of a coronary artery crossing the RV outflow tract (where the surgeon would like to work). The most common variants of concern are dual LADs and an LAD from the RCA with an anterior course. Significant or unusual conal branches also should be identified.

Conduits

There are a variety of cardiac malformations that require placement of a conduit to the pulmonary arteries (including TOF/PA). In these situations if intervention on the conduit is considered, it is necessary to assess the relationship

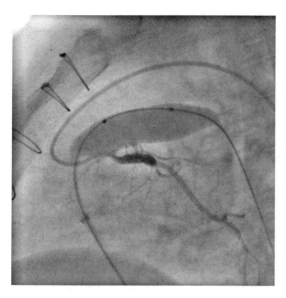

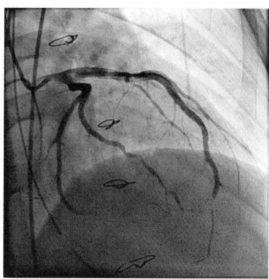

Fig. 9 Evaluation of the coronaries prior to RVOT stent placement

Fig. 10 Posttransplant coronary vasculopathy

of the coronary arteries to the conduit prior to intervention, because a conduit stent can easily compress a coronary artery (e.g., LAD from RCA), with expected results, Fig. 9. This is discussed further in the chapter on dilation and stenting of RV-PA conduits.

Posttransplant Vasculopathy

The vasculopathy of posttransplant coronary artery disease typically consists of concentric myointimal proliferation that often involves the entire length of the vessel, including intramyocardial branches, Fig. 10. Angiographically, coronary vasculopathy usually manifests as small, occasionally beaded vessels with tiny, short and sparse intramyocardial branches. Less often, discrete stenoses or filling defects are seen.

Complications

The most feared complication relates to injection of air or other obstructive material into the coronary artery, causing myocardial ischemia and possible infarction. This can be prevented by the

methods described above. Should an air embolus occur or should it be suspected, the patient should immediately be placed on 100% oxygen. There is a chance of altered hemodynamics and rhythm disturbances, both of which should be treated with aggressive supportive care. The patient should receive pain control or sedation if possible, to decrease myocardial oxygen consumption. Barring a large air embolus, nearly all patients should be able to be supported through the episode, without long-term sequelae. However, rare patients will proceed to cardiac arrest or myocardial infarction. The best treatment is prevention.

Coronary artery dissection is usually the result of forceful injection of contrast into a small side branch or a catheter directed against the side of a wall. Again, evidence of ischemia or rhythm disturbance can develop. Follow-up angiography may demonstrate a flap or extravasation.

Coronary artery spasm is often seen if the catheter tip has been advanced too far into the vessel. If this is recognized quickly and the catheter is pulled back, the spasm will usually self-resolve without necessary treatment. However, if the spasm persists or hemodynamic changes develop, the patient can be treated with an infusion of nitroglycerin directly into the vessel.

Appendix

Helpful General Equations and Information

1 French = 0.33 mm

1 cm H_2O = 0.7355 mmHg

1 atm = 760 mmHg

Cook Percutaneous-Entry Needle Sizes and Wires Accepted

	Gauge	Max Wire
Green	21 g	0.018″
Yellow	20 g	0.021″
Brown	19 g	0.035″
Pink	18 g	0.038″

Calibration [based on (empty) catheter size (1 Fr = 0.33 mm)]

F	mm	F	mm
3 F	1.0 mm	10 F	3.3 mm
4 F	1.3 mm	11 F	3.67 mm
5 F	1.7 mm	12 F	4.0 mm
6 F	2.0 mm	14 F	4.67 mm
7 F	2.3 mm	16 F	5.3 mm
8 F	2.67 mm	18 F	6.0 mm
9 F	3.0 mm	20 F	6.7 mm

Characteristics of Commonly Used Balloons

Tyshak® MINI (B. Braun Medical, Inc.)
Advantages:
- Very low profile

Disadvantages:
- Compliant
- Tiny wire
- Slow inflation/deflation
- Lower pressures in bigger balloons
- Limited size range

Common uses:
- Pulmonary valves in infants
- Newborns and infants

Tyshak-II (B. Braun Medical, Inc.)
Advantages:
- Low profile
- More stable larger wire than Tyshak®-MINI

Disadvantages:
- Compliant
- Slow inflation/deflation
- Lower pressures in bigger balloons

Common uses:
- Pulmonary valves in infants
- Newborns and infants

Symmetry™ (Boston Scientific Corporation)
Advantages:
- Very low profile
- Moderate pressures
- Hydrophilic coating for better tracking

Disadvantages:
- Limited size range
- Hydrophilic coating makes stent less stable on balloon

Common uses:
- Distal PA dilations
- Redilating small stents

Ultra-Thin™ Diamond (Boston Scientific Corporation)
Advantages:
- Relatively low profile
- Short taper
- Moderately high pressure
- Hydrophilic coating for better tracking

Disadvantages:
- Limited size range
- Hydrophilic coating makes stent less stable on balloon

Common uses:
- PA dilations

Ultra-thin SDS (Boston Scientific Corporation)
Advantages:
- Moderate pressures
- Noncompliant
- Short taper
- Puncture resistant
- "Holds" stent well

Disadvantages:
- Moderate profile
- Limited size range

Common uses:
- Stent placement
- PA dilation
- Valve dilations

Z-Med™ Balloon Dilation Catheters (B. Braun Medical, Inc.)
Advantages:
- Nice size range
- Short taper

Disadvantages:
- Moderate to low pressures
- High profile

Common uses:
- Proximal PA dilation

XXL™ (Boston Scientific Corporation)
Advantages:
- Moderate pressures
- Low profile for large balloons
- Nice size range for large balloons

Disadvantages:
- Long taper
- Not as good for placing stents
- Occasionally will not come out of a 7 sheath as specified

Common uses:
- Coarctation dilations
- Proximal PA dilation
- Aortic valve dilations

POWERFLEX™ P3 PTA Dilation Catheter and MAXI LD™ PTA Dilation Catheter (Cordis®)

Advantages:
  o Moderate pressures
  o Short taper
  o Decent profile for large balloons

Common uses:
  o Stent placement
  o Proximal PA dilation
  o Aortic valve dilations

CONQUEST™ and ATLAS® (Bard Peripheral Vascular, Inc.)

Advantages:
  o High pressure, puncture resistant

Disadvantages:
  o Relatively stiff body (poor tracking around curves)

Common uses:
  o Resistant stenosis, calcified conduits, stent redilations

Sizing Balloon

Advantages:
  o Very compliant

Common uses:
  o Sizing defects (septal and perivalvar)

Flexotome Cutting Balloon Device and Peripheral Cutting Balloon (Boston Scientific Corporation)

Advantages:
  o Controlled intimal/medial tear

Disadvantages:
  o Avoid in curved vessels

Common uses:
  o Resistant stenosis

Balloon Inventory Children's Hospital Boston, July 2008

Name	Diameter (mm)	Length (cm)	Sheath (F)	Wire	Max Pressure (ATM)	Shaft (cm)
Sub-4	2	2	4	18	15	90
Maverick	2.25	9	3.2	14	14	135
Maverick	2.5	9	3.2	14	14	135
Sub-4	2.5	2	4	18	15	90
Maverick	2.75	9	3.2	14	14	135
Maverick	3	9 mm, 2 cm	3.2	14	14	135
Sub-4	3	2	4	18	15	90
Ultrathin	3	2	5	35	15	120
Maverick	3.25	9 mm	3.2	14	14	135
Maverick	3.5	9 mm, 2 cm	3.2	14	12	135
Sub-4	3.5	2	4	18	15	90
Maverick	4	9 mm, 2 cm	3.2	14	12	135
Sub-4	4	2	4	18	15	90
Tyshak II	4	2	4	21	6	70
Ultrathin	4	2	5	35	15	120
Sub-4	4.5	2	5	18	15	90
Maverick	4.5	1.2, 2	3.2	14	18	135
Conquest	5	2	6	35	30	75
Sub-4	5	2	5	18	15	90
Maverick	5	2	4.2	14	18	135
Tyshak II	5	2	4	21	6	70
Tyshak Mini	5	2	3	14	6	65
Ultrathin	5	2	5	35	15	120
Ultrathin SDS	5	2	5	35	12	90
Conquest	5	4	6	35	30	75
Ultraverse	5	2	4	18	12	120
Sub-4	5.5	2	5	18	15	90
Conquest	6	2	6	35	30	75
Opti-Plast	6	2	5	35	12	100
Sub-4	6	2	5	18	15	90
Tyshak II	6	2	4	21	4	70
Tyshak Mini	6	2	3	14	4	65
Ultrathin	6	2	5	35	15	120
Ultrathin SDS	6	2	5	35	12	90
Ultraverse	6	2	5	18	12	120
Conquest	7	2	6	35	30	75
Opti-Plast	7	2	5	35	12	100
Sterling	7	2	4	14/18	14	80
Tyshak II	7	2	4	21	4	70
Tyshak Mini	7	2	3	14	4	65
Ultrathin	7	2	5	35	15	120
Ultrathin SDS	7	2	5	35	12	90
Ultraverse	7	2	5	18	12	120
Conquest	8	2	6	35	27	75
Opti-Plast	8	2	5	35	10	100
Sterling	8	2	4	14/18	12	80
Tyshak II	8	2	4	21	4	70
Ultrathin	8	2	6	35	15	120

(continued)

Name	Diameter (mm)	Length (cm)	Sheath (F)	Wire	Max Pressure (ATM)	Shaft (cm)
Ultrathin SDS	8	2	6	35	12	90
Tyshak MINI	8	2	3	14	4	65
Sub-4	9	2	7	35	12	90
Conquest	9	2	7	35	26	75
Sterling	9	2	5	14/18	10	80
Tyshak II	9	2	5	25	3.5	90
Conquest	9	4	7	35	26	75
Opti-Plast	9	2	6	35	9	100
Ultrathin	9	2	7	35	12	120
Ultrathin SDS	9	2	7	35	12	90
Conquest	10	2, 4	7	35	24	75
Opti-Plast	10	2	6	35	8	100
Sterling	10	2	5	14/18	10	80
Tyshak II	10	2	5	25	3.5	90
Sub-4	10	2, 3	7	35	12	90
Ultrathin	10	2	7	35	12	120
Ultrathin SDS	10	2, 3	7	35	12	90
Atlas	12	2, 4	7	35	18	120
Cordis	12	2, 4	7	35	8	110
Tyshak II	12	2	5	25	3.5	90
XXL	12	2, 4	7	35	8	120
Atlas	14	2, 4	7	35	18	120
Cordis	14	4	8	35	6	110
XXL	14	2, 4	7	35	8	120
Cordis	15	2, 4, 6	9	35	6	110
Atlas	16	2, 4	8	35	18	120
Cordis	16	4	10	35	6	110
XXL	16	2, 4	7	35	5	120
Atlas	18	2, 4	8	35	16	120
Cordis	18	4, 6	10	35	6	110
XXL	18	2, 4	8	35	5	120
Atlas	20	2, 4	9	35	16	120
Cordis	20	4, 6	11	35	6	110
Z-Med II	20	4, 5	12	35	5	100
ATLAS	22	2, 4	10	35	14	75
Z-Med II	22	4	12	35	4	100
ATLAS	24	2, 4	10	35	14	75
Z-Med (non II)	25	4	12	35	3	100
Z-Med	26	4	12	35	3	100
ATLAS	26	2, 4	12	35	12	75
Z-Med	28	4	12	35	2	85
Z-Med II	30	5	16	35	3	100
Z-Med	30	4	14	35	2	85

Balloon Inventory Children's Hospital Boston, October 2007

Name	Diameter (mm)	Length (cm)	Sheath (F)	Wire	Max Pressure (ATM)	Shaft (cm)
Sizing Balloons						
Numed	20	3	8	35	1.5	80
Numed	25	3	8	35	1.5	80
Numed	30	3	8	35	1.0	80
Numed	40	3	9	35	0.5	80
Cutting Balloons						
Cutting Balloon	2.0	1	5	14	12	137
Cutting Balloon	2.5	1	5	14	12	137
Cutting Balloon	2.75	1	6	.014	12	137
Cutting Balloon	2	1.5	6	.014	12	140
Cutting Balloon	3	1.5	6	.014	12	140
Cutting Balloon	4	1.5	6	.014	12	140
Cutting Balloon	3.0	1	5	14	12	137
Cutting Balloon	3.5	1	5	14	12	137
Cutting Balloon	4.0	1	5	14	12	137
Cutting Balloon	5	2	7	18	10	90
Cutting Balloon	6	2	7	18	10	90
Cutting Balloon	7	2	7	18	10	90
Cutting Balloon	8	2	7	18	10	90

Approved Devices

CardioSEAL (NMT Medical, Inc.)

Size (mm)	Sheath (Fr)
17	10
23	10
28	10
33	10
40	12

AMPLATZER Duct Occluder (AGA Medical Corporation)

Aorta (A)	PA (B)	Length (D)	Retention Skirt (C)	Sheath (Fr)
5	4	5	9	6
6	4	7	10	6
8	6	7	12	7
10	8	8	16	7
12	10	8	18	7

AMPLATZER Vascular Plug (AGA Medical Corporation)

Size (mm)	Length (mm)	Sheath (Fr)
4	7	5*
6	7	5*
8	7	5*
10	7	6
12	8	6
14	8	8
16	8	8

* May also be inserted via a large-lumen coronary catheter.

AMPLATZER Septal Occluder

Size (mm)	LA diam (mm)	RA diam (mm)	Sheath (Fr)
4	+12	+8	6
5	+12	+8	6
6	+12	+8	6
7	+12	+8	6
8	+12	+8	6
9	+12	+8	6
10	+12	+8	6
11	+14	+10	7
12	+14	+10	7
13	+14	+10	7
14	+14	+10	7
15	+14	+10	7
16	+14	+10	7
17	+14	+10	7
18	+14	+10	8
19	+14	+10	8
20	+14	+10	8
22	+14	+10	9
24	+14	+10	9
26	+14	+10	10
28	+14	+10	10
30	+14	+10	10
32	+14	+10	12
34	+16	+10	12
36	+16	+10	12
38	+16	+10	12

Angiographic Catheter Volumes
and Flow Rates

Pigtail Catheters

Manufacturer	Size (F)	Length (cm)	Max Injection (cc/sec)
Merit	3	40	5
Merit	3	50	4
Merit	4	50	13
Merit	4	80	10
Cook	4	70	20
Merit	5	100	18
Merit	5	80	20
Cook	5	100	27
Merit	6	80	35
Merit	6	100	31
Merit	7	100	42

Berman Angiographic Balloon Catheter ARROW® (Arrow International, Inc.)

Size (F)	Length (cm)	Max Injection (cc/sec)
4	50	5
5	50	15
5	80	12
7	90	22

Soft-Vu® Halo™ (AngioDynamics, Inc.)

Size (F)	Length (cm)	Max Injection (cc/sec)
4	65	20
5	65	33

BSA Chart

Pt Height (in)	Pt Height (cm)	Pt Weight (lb)	Pt Weight (kg)	BSA (Dubois)	BSA (Haycock)
66	167.64	300	136.05	2.38	2.60
66	167.64	290	131.52	2.34	2.55
66	167.64	280	126.98	2.31	2.50
66	167.64	270	122.45	2.27	2.45
66	167.64	260	117.91	2.24	2.40
66	167.64	250	113.38	2.20	2.35
66	167.64	240	108.84	2.16	2.30
66	167.64	230	104.31	2.12	2.25
66	167.64	220	99.77	2.08	2.20
66	167.64	210	95.24	2.04	2.14
66	167.64	200	90.70	2.00	2.09
66	167.64	190	86.17	1.96	2.03
66	167.64	180	81.63	1.91	1.97
66	167.64	170	77.10	1.87	1.91
66	167.64	160	72.56	1.82	1.85
66	167.64	150	68.03	1.77	1.79
66	167.64	140	63.49	1.72	1.72
66	167.64	130	58.96	1.67	1.66
66	167.64	120	54.42	1.61	1.59
66	167.64	110	49.89	1.55	1.51
66	167.64	100	45.35	1.49	1.44
36	91.44	100	45.35	0.96	1.13
36	91.44	90	40.82	0.92	1.07
36	91.44	80	36.28	0.87	1.00
36	91.44	70	31.75	0.82	0.93
36	91.44	60	27.21	0.77	0.86
36	91.44	50	22.68	0.71	0.78
36	91.44	40	18.14	0.65	0.69
36	91.44	30	13.61	0.58	0.59
36	91.44	20	9.07	0.48	0.48
36	91.44	10	4.54	0.36	0.33
36	91.44	0	0.00	0.00	0.00

Oxygen Consumption Charts

Oxygen Consumption per Body Surface Area[*]

Age (yr)	Heart Rate (beats/min)												
	50	60	70	80	90	100	110	120	130	140	150	160	170
Male Patients													
3				155	159	163	167	171	175	178	182	186	190
4			149	152	156	160	163	168	171	175	179	182	186
6		141	144	148	151	155	159	162	167	171	174	178	181
8		136	141	145	148	152	156	159	163	167	171	175	178
10	130	134	139	142	146	149	153	157	160	165	169	172	176
12	128	132	136	140	144	147	151	155	158	162	167	170	174
14	127	130	134	137	142	146	149	153	157	160	165	169	172
16	125	129	132	136	141	144	148	152	155	159	162	167	
18	124	127	131	135	139	143	147	150	154	157	161	166	
20	123	126	130	134	137	142	145	149	153	156	160	165	
25	120	124	127	131	135	139	143	147	150	154	157		
30	118	122	125	129	133	136	141	145	148	152	155		
35	116	120	124	127	131	135	139	143	147	150			
40	115	119	122	126	130	133	137	141	145	149			

[*]In (mL/min)/m^2. From LaFarge CG, Miettinen OS: The estimation of oxygen consumption. *Cardiovasc Res* 4:23, 1970. Taken from Park, MK: *Pediatric Cardiology for Practitioners*, 4th ed. Copyright © 2002 Mosby, Inc.

Oxygen Consumption per Body Surface Area[*]

Age (yr)	Heart Rate (beats/min)												
	50	60	70	80	90	100	110	120	130	140	150	160	170
Female Patients													
3				150	153	157	161	165	169	172	176	180	183
4			141	145	149	152	156	159	163	168	171	175	179
6		130	134	137	142	146	149	153	156	160	165	168	172
8		125	129	133	136	141	144	148	152	155	159	163	167
10	118	122	125	129	133	136	141	144	148	152	155	159	163
12	115	119	122	126	130	133	137	141	145	149	152	156	160
14	112	116	120	123	127	131	134	138	143	146	150	153	157
16	109	114	118	121	125	128	132	136	140	144	148	151	
18	107	111	116	119	123	127	130	134	137	142	146	149	
20	106	109	114	118	121	125	128	132	136	140	144	148	
25	102	106	109	114	118	121	125	128	132	136	140		
30	99	103	106	110	115	118	122	125	129	133	136		
35	97	100	104	107	111	116	119	123	127	130			
50	94	98	102	105	109	112	117	121	124	128			

[*]In (mL/min)/m^2. From LaFarge CG, Miettinen OS: The estimation of oxygen consumption. *Cardiovasc Res* 4:23, 1970. Taken from Park, MK: *Pediatric Cardiology for Practitioners*, 4th ed. Copyright © 2002 Mosby, Inc.

Effective Dilating Diameter (mm) Using
Double Balloon Technique

	6 mm	7 mm	8 mm	10 mm	12 mm	14 mm	15 mm	16 mm	18 mm	20 mm	22 mm	24 mm
6 mm	9.0											
7 mm	10.7	11.5										
8 mm	11.5	12.3	13.1									
10 mm	13.3	14.0	14.8	16.4								
12 mm	15.1	15.8	16.5	18.0	19.6							
14 mm	16.9	17.6	18.3	19.7	21.3	22.9						
15 mm	17.8	18.5	19.2	20.6	22.1	23.7	24.5					
16 mm	18.7	19.4	20.1	21.5	23.0	24.6	25.4	26.2				
18 mm	20.6	21.2	21.9	23.3	24.7	26.3	27.0	27.8	29.5			
20 mm	22.5	23.1	23.7	25.1	26.5	28.0	28.8	29.5	31.1	32.7		
22 mm	24.4	25.0	25.6	26.9	28.3	29.7	30.5	31.2	32.8	34.4	36.0	
24 mm	26.3	26.9	27.5	28.8	30.1	31.5	32.2	33.0	34.5	36.1	37.7	39.3

Yeager SB. Balloon selection for double balloon valvotomy. *J Am Coll Cardiol* 1987;9:467–468.

Abbreviations

aAo	ascending aorta
ACT	activated clotting time
ADO	AMPLATZER ductal occluder
ALCAPA	anomalous left coronary artery from the pulmonary artery
Ao	aorta
AODT	descending thoracic aorta
AoV	aortic valve
APC	aorto-pulmonary collateral
AR	aortic regurgitation
AS	aortic stenosis
ASA	atrial septal aneurysm
ASD	atrial septal defect
ASO	AMPLATZER septal occluder
ATM	atmosphere
BAS	balloon atrial septostomy
BDG	bi-directional Glenn
BIB	balloon-in-balloon
BPD	bronchopulmonary dysplasia
BSA	body surface area
BTS	Blalock–Tausig shunt
CHD	congenital heart disease
CI	cardiac Index
Circ/Cx	circumflex coronary artery
CO	cardiac output
CoA	coarctation of the aorta
CS	coronary sinus
CVA	cerebrovascular accidents
CXR	chest X-ray
dAo	descending aorta
EDP	end diastolic pressure
EJV	external jugular vein
EMB	endomyocardial biopsy
EP	electrophysiology
FA	femoral artery
Hct	hematocrit
HLHS	hypoplastic left heart syndrome
HTN	hypertension
ICE	intracardiac echocardiogram
IJV	internal jugular vein
IVC	inferior vena cava
IVS	intact ventricular septum
JR	Judkins right
LA	left atrium
LAD	left anterior descending coronary artery
LAO	long axial oblique
LAp	left atrial pressure
LCA/ LMCA	left main coronary artery
LFV	left femoral vein
LPA	left pulmonary artery
LPCWp	left pulmonary capillary wedge pressure
LSVC	left superior vena cava
LUPV	left upper pulmonary vein

(continued)

LV	left ventricle
LVED	left ventricle end diastole
LVEDp	left ventricle end diastolic pressure
LVH	left ventricle hypertrophy
MPA	main pulmonary artery
MR	mitral regurgitation
MS	mitral stenosis
MV	mitral valve
OHT	orthotopic heart transplant
PA	pulmonary artery
PA/IVS	pulmonary atresia with intact ventricular septum
PAp	pulmonary artery pressure
PAPVR	partial anomalous pulmonary venous return
PBF	Pulmonary blood flow
PCWP	pulmonary capillary wedge pressure
PDA	posterior descending coronary artery
PFO	patent foramen ovale
PGE	prostaglandin E1
PR	pulmonary regurgitation
PS	pulmonary stenosis
PV	pulmonary valve
PVR	pulmonary vascular resistance
PVWp	pulmonary venous wedge pressure
Qp	pulmonary flow
Qs	systemic flow
RA	right atrium
RAO	right anterior oblique
RAp	right atrial pressure
RCA	right coronary artery
RF	radiofrequency
RFCA	radiofrequency ablation
RFV	right femoral vein
RIJV	right internal jugular vein
RPA	right pulmonary artery
RPCWp	right pulmonary capillary wedge pressure
RSCV	right subclavian vein
RUPV	right upper pulmonary vein
RV	right ventricle
RVDCC	right ventricle dependant coronary circulation
RVEDp	right ventricle end diastolic pressure
RVOT	right ventricle outflow tract
RVOTO	right ventricle outflow tract obstruction
RVp	right ventricular pressure
RV/PA	right ventricle-to-pulmonary artery
RVVO	right ventricle volume overload
SCV	subclavian vein
SVC	superior vena cava
SVT	supraventricular tachycardia
TEE	transesophageal echocardiogram
TGA	transposition of the great arteries
TOF	Tetralogy of Fallot
TOF/PA	Tetralogy of Fallot with pulmonary artery atresia
TR	tricuspid regurgitation
TV	tricuspid valve
US	ultrasound
VSD	ventricular septal defect

Index

The page numbers with letter '*f*' denotes figures (For example 28*f* denotes figure in page number 28)
The page numbers with letter '*t*' denotes tables. (For example 46*t* denotes table in page number 46)